T0100198

EBOLA VIRUS DISEASE (EVD)

OUTBREAKS, CONTROL AND PREVENTION STRATEGIES

VIROLOGY RESEARCH PROGRESS

Additional books and e-books in this series can be found on Nova's website under the Series tab.

VIROLOGY RESEARCH PROGRESS

EBOLA VIRUS DISEASE (EVD)

OUTBREAKS, CONTROL AND PREVENTION STRATEGIES

HILAIRE VERREAU
EDITOR

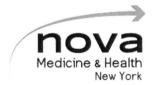

Medicine & Health
New York

NOTICE TO THE READER

Library of Congress Cataloging-in-Publication Data

ISBN: 978-1-53616-291-2

Published by Nova Science Publishers, Inc. † *New York*

CONTENTS

Contents

PREFACE

To mitigate the spread of the rare and deadly disease Ebola, Ebola Virus Disease (EVD): Outbreaks, Control and Prevention Strategies begins with the proposition of a mathematical model with vital dynamics and two preventive measures: quarantine and isolation.

Humanitarian issues in Ebola prevention and control are explored, as well as the cultural practices and social norms during outbreaks. Additionally, some innovative approaches in the humanitarian response to prevention and control are discussed.

The authors expose the dilemma Ebola poses to within the healthcare system, where healthcare providers are caught between the over-arching quest for self-preservation from a highly virulent disease and the professional demand of prioritising the interests of the patients over self.

In conclusion, the authors describe successfully developed drug candidates from their laboratory for the treatment Ebola using EBOV protein structure, such as VP24, VP35, VP40, nucleoprotein, and glycoprotein.

Chapter 1 - To mitigate the spread of the rare and deadly disease Ebola, the authors propose a mathematical model with vital dynamics and two preventive measures: quarantine and isolation. The model parameters are estimated using the method of Least Squares, the chain of posteriors is computed, and posteriors mean compared with estimates from the Least

Squares method. The basic reproduction number is $R_0 = 2.79$. To reduce
simulation uncertainties due to potential inaccuracy from model parameter
values, the Markov Chain Monte Carlo method is applied to improve
model parameter estimates and the simulation accuracy.

Chapter 2 - At present, there is no vaccine against Ebola Virus
suggesting a stalemate in man's effort to curb this extremely fatal disease.
This life-threatening scenario implies that prevention and control measure
of Ebola Virus Disease (EVD) are predominantly centered on case
identification and isolation, early broad-based medical care, surveillance of
suspected cases, and safe burial practices. Optimizing the existing control
and prevention strategies such as community engagement and awareness,
improved access to personal protective equipment (PPE), Community Care
Centers (CCC) and EVD treatment (if any) are pivotal in the prevention
and control strategy. The preliminary key to a successful outbreak control
is hinged on community engagement by creating awareness to risk factors
and prevention measures. The importance of vaccine to combat the disease
is also highlighted. The chapter also discussed humanitarian issues in EVD
prevention and control and humanitarian protection during EVD outbreak
and the challenges posed by cultural practices and social norms during
outbreaks. Some innovative approaches in the humanitarian response to
prevention and control have been discussed.

Chapter 3 - The persons infected with Ebola Virus Disease (EVD) are
victims of a wide range of constraints to their human rights as protected by
law. Such persons' rights are often violated because of their presumed or
known EVD status, causing them to suffer both the burden of the disease
and the social burden of discrimination and stigmatisation which could
deter the infected persons from accessing available treatment. The victims
failure or reluctance to avail themselves for treatment invariably
contributes to the spreading of the disease. The work further exposes the
dilemma posed by the EVD to the healthcare system, where healthcare
providers are caught between the over-arching quest for self-preservation
from a highly virulent disease and the professional demand of prioritising
the interests of their patients over self.

Chapter 4 - Ebola disease is an acute fever disease that is caused by infection of viruses within the genus *Ebolavirus* such as *Zaire ebolavirus, Sudan ebolavirus, Bundibugyo ebolavirus, Taï Forest ebolavirus,* and *Reston ebolavirus.* Almost all species cause disease in human, except *Reston ebolavirus* which is only known to cause disease in nonhuman primates. Ebola infection in human has similar initial symptoms with influenza or malaria which are marked with pyrexia, sore head, muscle or joint pain, weakness, vomiting, abdomen pain, as well as bleeding. The virus can spread by direct contact from human to human through various bodily fluids such as saliva, blood, stool, semen, breast milk, and tears. Ebola virus proteins comprise of non-structural proteins, nucleoprotein, matrix protein, and glycoproteins. Since its discovery in 1976, Ebola virus has become an epidemic in the African continent. The most extensive Ebola case in history was confirmed at the end of March 2016 with 11,325 deaths in West Africa. Unfortunately, there is no FDA-approved drug to treat this viral infection in human. Drug discovery and development for EVD is a complex process which requires a long time, many resources, and huge capital. Because of that, another approach has to apply in order to reduce all of the necessities. Bioinformatics studies through the Computer-Aided Drug Design (CADD) method can be employed to find the potential drug candidates at the preliminary stage of drug discovery. The authors' research group has successfully developed drug candidates to treat Ebola by using EBOV protein structure. Most of these drug candidates were obtained from some free online databases and were processed through molecular docking simulation. The drug candidates which was selected must comply with the requirements such as attaching to the binding sites of the protein, have energy binding value lower than standards, and exhibited preferable interaction with the protein. The screening process also involves pharmacokinetics analysis and toxicity prediction by using software to suppress possible failure when evaluated later in the wet laboratory. In this chapter, the authors describe the successful developed drug candidates from their laboratory to treat Ebola by using EBOV protein structure, such as VP24, VP35, VP40, nucleoprotein, and glycoprotein.

In: Ebola Virus Disease (EVD)   ISBN: 978-1-53616-291-2
Editor: Hilaire Verreau   © 2019 Nova Science Publishers, Inc.

Chapter 1

MODELLING THE DISTRIBUTION AND SPREAD OF EBOLA DISEASE IN WEST AFRICA

Denis Ndanguza[1]*, PhD, J. de Dieu Niyigena*[1]*, MD
and Jean M. Tchuenche*[2]*, PhD*

[1] Department of Mathematics, College of Science and Technology,
University of Rwanda, Kigali, Rwanda
[2] School of Computer Science and Applied Mathematics,
University of the Witwatersrand, Johannesburg, South Africa

Abstract

To mitigate the spread of the rare and deadly disease Ebola, we propose a mathematical model with vital dynamics and two preventive measures: quarantine and isolation. The model parameters are estimated using the method of Least Squares, the chain of posteriors is computed, and posteriors mean compared with estimates from the Least Squares method. The basic reproduction number is $R_0 = 2.79$. To reduce simulation uncertainties due to potential inaccuracy from model parameter values, the Markov Chain Monte Carlo method is applied to improve model parameter estimates and the simulation accuracy.

Keywords: Ebola, spatial distribution, preventive measures, posteriors

---

*Corresponding Author's Email: dndanguza@gmail.com

1.   Introduction

Mathematical models play an important role in assessing the potential impact of prevention and control strategies of infectious diseases, and can help derive set of conditions through quantification of interventions prior to their implementation; thereby providing stakeholders (e.g., policy makers, the media, healthcare personnel, and the public) with appropriate, quantifiable evidence to support decision making (Rivers et al., 2014). This in turn, provides policy makers, the media, healthcare personnel, and the public with appropriate, quantifiable evidence to support decision making (Rivers et al., 2014).

Ebola virus disease (EVD also referred to as Ebola hemorrhagic fever – EHF), or simply Ebola, is a disease of humans and other primates. The virus spreads by direct contact (through broken skin or mucous membranes) with the blood, organs, secretions or other bodily fluids (stool, urine, saliva, semen) of an infected human or other animals, and upon contact with a recently contaminated item or surface. Local burial customs where dead bodies are washed before burial can also contribute to transmission. Men who have recovered from Ebola are said to transmit the virus (up to 7 weeks after recovery) to their partner through semen. Breastfeeding is also a risk factor[1] as babies may acquire the virus through breast milk of infected mothers (CDC, 2016). Signs and symptoms typically start between two days and three weeks after contracting the virus as a fever, sore throat, muscle pain, and headaches. The 2014 outbreak of the Ebola virus disease has shown how quickly diseases can spread in human populations and health officials need to make quick and informed decisions as how to mitigate the high burden of this disease. Control of outbreaks requires coordinated medical services, alongside a certain level of community engagement. For this reason, mathematical modeling importance cannot be overemphasized. It provides long-term impact of interventions and a key tool when field and laboratory data are not available.

---

[1]Ebola also appears in the breast milk of infected women after recovery, and the time taken for it to disappear is not known (CDC, 2016).

Ebola is the most spread epidemic[2] of the Ebola Virus Disease (EVD). The EVD history can be traced back to the Democratic Republic of Congo (formerly Zaïre) and Sudan in the year 1976 (CDC, 2016). Although the origin of the Ebola virus is unknown, little evidence has emerged indicating that forest animals such as fruit bats, chimpanzees, gorillas, monkeys, forest antelope and porcupines are hosts of the Ebola virus (Legrand et al., 2007).

On June 2016, the World Health Organization (WHO) reported a total of 28,616 Ebola cases, with Sierra Leone and Guinea leading in transmission. During the 2014 outbreak, 3,814 and 14,124 occurred in Guinea and Sierra Leone respectively with 2,544 and 3,956 deaths. Liberia registered a total of 10,678 cases of which, 4,810 died during the same period. The epidemic spread to other African countries such as Nigeria (20 cases), Senegal (1 case), and Mali (8 cases) as well as to some non-African countries: One Ebola case occurred in Spain and in the United Kingdom, and four cases occurred in United States (CDC, 2016).

The Ebola virus disease is transmitted via direct contact (through broken skin or mucous membranes) with the blood, organs, secretions or other bodily fluids (stool, urine, saliva, semen) of infected people. Surfaces and materials such as beddings, and clothing contaminated with body fluids of infected people, local burial customs where dead bodies are washed before burial can also contribute to transmission. Men who have recovered from Ebola are said to transmit the virus (up to 7 weeks after recovery) to their partner through semen. Breastfeeding is also a risk factor[3] as babies may acquire the virus through breast milk of infected mothers (CDC, 2016). Symptoms of Ebola are divided into two stages: The first stage often includes fever, headache, sore throat, fatigue, and muscle pain. This stage can often be mistaken for other diseases such as malaria or typhoid. The second stage includes more severe symptoms such as vomiting, diarrhoea, rash and in some cases, internal and external bleeding. Recovery is more likely to occur from the first stage, with much higher death rates in the second stage (indeed, in some outbreaks all second-stage patients die). Ebola is unlikely to be transmitted during the incubation period and the

---

[2]A disease is epidemic if it spreads rapidly to a large number of people in a given population of a particular region within a short period of time (Newman, 2002).

[3]Ebola also appears in the breast milk of infected women after recovery, and the time taken for it to disappear is not known (CDC, 2016).

transmissibility is likely to be higher as the disease progresses. An Ebola patient can take from 2 weeks to 2 months to recover from the time she/he gets the symptoms (CDC, 2016).

Although there are currently no marketable vaccines or drugs for Ebola, several prevention and control measures are available. Prevention strategies targeted at reducing contact between people at risk and those infected have been supported by governments and the world at large. These include wearing appropriate personal protective equipments (PPE), practice proper infection control, isolating patients with Ebola from other patients, and avoiding direct or unprotected contact with the bodies of people who have died from Ebola. In addition, it is strongly requested to notify health officials when direct contact with infected individuals occurs (CDC, 2016).

Mathematical models of the transmission dynamics of Ebola abound in the literature (Chowell et al., 2004; Legrand et al., 2007; Banton et al., 2010; Ndanguza et al., 2013; Bashar et al., 2014; Camacho et al., 2014; Salaam-Blyther, 2014; Rivers et al., 2014; Lewnard et al., 2014; Khan et al., 2015; Yamin et al., 2015; Agusto et al., 2015; Barbarossa et al., 2015; Webb and Browne, 2016; Berge et al., 2017) and the references therein. We refine the model proposed in Ndanguza et al. (2013) to include both isolation (separating those individuals who are sick from those who are not to reduce transmission of the disease) and quarantine (separating those who may have been exposed to the disease until they either show signs of the disease or are no longer a risk). Indeed, implementing a combined approach of case isolation, contact-tracing with quarantine is important to stem the rapid growth of Ebola outbreak (Yi et al., 2009). Quarantine, also known as enforced isolation, is usually effective in decreasing disease spread (Hethcote et al., 2002). Over the centuries quarantine has been used to reduce the transmission of human diseases such as leprosy, plague, cholera, typhus, yellow fever, smallpox, diphtheria, tuberculosis, measles, mumps, ebola and lassa fever (Hethcote, 2000; Hethcote et al., 2002).

For an outbreak of a disease such as Ebola, where no prescribed or recommended therapeutic interventions are available, isolation of diagnosed infectives and quarantine of individuals who might have been infected (usually by contact-tracing of diagnosed infectives) are the only two potentially realistic control measures available. The novelty of this study is the inclusion of these two population classes (that were missing in the model proposed by Ndanguza et al. (2013) and Chowell et al. (2004).

The rest of the chapter is organized as follows: Section 2 is the model formulation. Section 3 provides the description of the model parameters estimation using least square method. The stability of the disease-free equilibrium is investigated in Section 4 as well as the computation of the model basic reproduction number. In Section 5, numerical simulations are provided to support the theoretical results. The conclusion is provided in Section 6.

2. Model Formulation

The proposed model is an extension of Ndanguza et al. (2013) in which the total population is subdivided into eight classes based on individual's disease status: Susceptible (S), capable of contracting the disease; Exposed (E), infected with the disease but in a latent state (group of people who have been in contact with an infected individual or the pathogen/infectious agent); Quarantine (Q), to limit the contact rate of individuals from the E-class (after certain time, individuals who are positive move to the I class while those who are negative to the infectious agent move to the S-Class); infectious (I), class of individuals capable of infecting others (three possibilities may arise: to recover, to be isolated or to die); isolated (J), infectious and diagnosed (isolated for intensive treatment-hospitalized and limitation with external contacts), isolated members leave the isolated class at rate of ω_1 if recovered and ω_2 if they die; recovered (R), group of individuals who eventually recover from the disease and dead (D), represents individuals who eventually succumb to the disease. It is assumed that not all dead individuals are buried (B). We assume that burial are carried out at a rate α. Also, we assume there is no transfer from the R class back to the S class, however, recovered individuals are under surveillance until the end of outbreak as it was the case in the recent West Africa Ebola outbreak. Since a proportion of susceptible individuals will be in contact with the dead, it is assumed that the latter could be infected at a rate ρ. Based on the model description and assumptions above, the refined model is represented diagrammatically in Figure 1.

The model variables are $S(t), E(t), Q(t), I(t), R(t), D(t), J(t)$ and $B(t)$, while the model parameters are given and defined below.

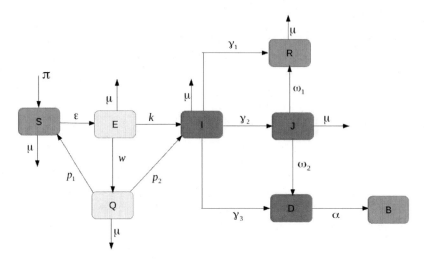

Figure 1. Flow diagram for the Ebola model.

- β_0 is the contact rate before intervention (in days),

- β_1 is the contact rate after intervention (in days),

- q stands for the rate from β_0 to β_1,

- $1/k$ is the incubation rate (in days),

- $1/\gamma_1$ is the disease recovery rate (in days),

- $1/\gamma_2$ is the removal rate from I to J (in days),

- $1/\gamma_3$ is the disease-related death rate when in I (in days),

- τ is the time at which interventions start (in days),

- ω_1 is the recovery rate when in J (in days^{-1}),

- ω_2 is the disease-related death rate when in J (in days^{-1}),

- p_1 is the immigration rate from Q to S (in days^{-1}),

- p_2 is the infectious rate from Q (in days^{-1}),

- w is the per capita rate of immigration from E to Q (in days^{-1}),

- μ is the death rate due to other diseases,

- π is the recruitment or birth rate,

- α is the burial ratio for dead bodies,

- ρ is the contact rate between susceptible and dead bodies,

- $\varepsilon = \frac{S(t)}{N}(\beta(t)I(t) + \rho D(t))$ is called standard incidence.

Based on our model flow diagram, descriptions and assumptions, we establish the following system of nonlinear ordinary equations (ODEs).

$$
\begin{aligned}
\frac{dS(t)}{dt} &= \pi - \frac{S(t)}{N}(\beta(t)I(t) + \rho D(t)) + p_1 Q(t) - \mu S(t), \\[2mm]
\frac{dE(t)}{dt} &= \frac{S(t)}{N}(\beta(t)I(t) + \rho D(t)) - (k + w + \mu)E(t), \\[2mm]
\frac{dI(t)}{dt} &= kE(t) + p_2 Q(t) - (\gamma_1 + \gamma_2 + \gamma_3 + \mu)I(t), \\[2mm]
\frac{dR(t)}{dt} &= \gamma_1 I(t) + \omega_1 J(t) - \mu R(t), \\[2mm]
\frac{dD(t)}{dt} &= \gamma_3 I(t) + \omega_2 J(t) - \alpha D(t), \\[2mm]
\frac{dQ(t)}{dt} &= wE(t) - (p_1 + p_2 + \mu)Q(t), \\[2mm]
\frac{dJ(t)}{dt} &= \gamma_2 I(t) - (\omega_1 + \omega_2 + \mu)J(t), \\[2mm]
\frac{dB(t)}{dt} &= \alpha D(t).
\end{aligned}
\tag{1}
$$

with the contact rate formulated in Ndanguza et al. (2013) as

$$\beta(t) = \beta_0 + (\beta_1 - \beta_0) / \left(1 + e^{-q(t-\tau)}\right).$$ (2)

3. Estimation of Parameters Using Least Squares Method

Model parameter estimation is quite interesting as could be a daunting task, because this could prove to be computationally too expensive especially for large systems. This has led to the application of a technique determining which parameters affect the system's dynamics the most (Hamby, 1994). Model results can be highly correlated with an input parameter so that small changes in the input value result in significant changes in the output (Hamby, 1994). Sensitivity analysis is a subjective method (Downing et al., 1985) in the sense that it is simple and only qualitative; it often relies on experts' opinion to determine, a priori, which parameters can be discarded due to lack of influence on model results. However, one advantage of this method is that, for large models, where most other methods are impractical, the subjective method can be used as a first cut to reduce the number of input parameters to a manageable size (Hamby, 1994).

Although the Ebola model (1) includes many parameters, based on our sensitivity analysis, we have identified and selected twelve most sensitive parameters in this study $(\beta_0, \beta_1, k, \gamma_1, \gamma_2, \gamma_3, \omega_1, \omega_2, p_1, p_2, w, \alpha)$ because they are considered the most critical factors controlling the spread of Ebola.

Parameters described in System (1) are estimated using synthetic data generated by adding noise on deterministic solution of (1) by least-squares fit. This consists of minimizing the likelihood function which is the residual sum of squares (*RSS*).

$$RSS = \sum_{i=1}^{n} (Y_i - f(Y_i, \theta))^2,$$

where Y_i are generated data, $f(Y_i, \theta)$ is the model and θ the parameters to be estimated. For further literature on optimization and measure of model fit see (Ndanguza et al., 2013; Demiris, 2004; Robert and Casella, 2004; Morgan, 2000).

Assuming that at the beginning of the outbreak, there was one exposed individual $E_0 = 1; I_0 = 0; R_0 = 0; D_0 = 0; Q_0 = 0; J_0 = 0$ and $B_0 = 1$, means that $S_0 = 19999998$ (the entire population of West African countries affected by Ebola was approximately 20000000 during the outbreak period). Consulting (Chowell et al., 2004; Lekone and Finkenstadt, 2006), some initial parameters values are set following different constraints, others are assumed. Parameter estimates are listed in Table 1.

Table 1. Estimated Ebola epidemic model parameters using synthetic data by LSQ method

Parameters	Initial values	Estimates
β_0	8.2624	8.2953
β_1	0.0187	0.0188
$1/k$	3.248	3.2419
$1/\gamma_1$	8.2281	8.2925
$1/\gamma_2$	8.1921	8.2562
$1/\gamma_3$	3.6946	3.7235
ω_1	0.0521	0.0525
ω_2	0.0112	0.0113
p_1	0.0107	0.0106
p_2	0.0938	0.0945
w	0.2707	0.2728
α	0.7593	0.7225

4.   Qualitative Analysis

4.1.   Disease-Free Equilibrium

The computation of the disease free equilibrium is done after changing the scale (without N)

$$
\begin{aligned}
S' &= \pi - S(t)\left(\beta(t)I(t) + \rho D(t)\right) + p_1 Q(t) - \mu S(t), \\[4pt]
E' &= S(t)\left(\beta(t)I(t) + \rho D(t)\right) - (k + w + \mu)E(t), \\[4pt]
I' &= kE(t) + p_2 Q(t) - (\gamma_1 + \gamma_2 + \gamma_3 + \mu)I(t), \\[4pt]
R' &= \gamma_1 I(t) + \omega_1 J(t) - \mu R(t), \\[4pt]
D' &= \gamma_3 I(t) + \omega_2 J(t) - \alpha D(t), \\[4pt]
Q' &= wE(t) - (p_1 + p_2 + \mu)Q(t), \\[4pt]
J' &= \gamma_2 I(t) - (\omega_1 + \omega_2 + \mu)J(t), \\[4pt]
B' &= \alpha D(t).
\end{aligned}
\tag{3}
$$

Then we take $S' = E' = I' = R' = D' = Q' = J' = B' = 0$. The disease-free equilibrium is given by $E_0 = (\pi/\mu, 0, 0, 0, 0, 0, 0, 0) = (1, 0, 0, 0, 0, 0, 0, 0)$. We want to study the stability of the system around the disease free equilibrium E_0 by computing the Jacobian matrix and then find the eigenvalues.

Consider

$$f_1 = \pi - S(t)(\beta(t)I(t) + \rho D(t)) + p_1 Q(t) - \mu S(t),$$

$$f_2 = S(t)(\beta(t)I(t) + \rho D(t)) - (k + w + \mu)E(t)$$

$$f_3 = kE(t) + p_2 Q(t) - (\gamma_1 + \gamma_2 + \gamma_3 + \mu)I(t),$$

$$f_4 = \gamma_1 I(t) + \omega_1 J(t) - \mu R(t),$$

$$f_5 = \gamma_3 I(t) + \omega_2 J(t) - \alpha D(t),$$

$$f_6 = wE(t) - (p_1 + p_2 + \mu)Q(t),$$

$$f_7 = \gamma_2 I(t) - (\omega_1 + \omega_2 + \mu)J(t),$$

$$f_8 = \alpha D(t),$$

then the Jacobian matrix evaluated at E_0 will be

$$J_0 = \begin{pmatrix}
-\mu & 0 & -\beta_0 & 0 & -\rho & p_1 & 0 & 0 \\
0 & -(k+\mu+w) & \beta_0 & 0 & \rho & 0 & 0 & 0 \\
0 & k & -(\gamma_1+\gamma_2+\gamma_3+\mu) & 0 & 0 & p_2 & 0 & 0 \\
0 & 0 & \gamma_1 & -\mu & 0 & 0 & \omega_1 & 0 \\
0 & 0 & \gamma_3 & 0 & -\alpha & 0 & \omega_2 & 0 \\
0 & w & 0 & 0 & 0 & -(\mu+p_1+p_2) & 0 & 0 \\
0 & 0 & \gamma_2 & 0 & 0 & 0 & -(\mu+\omega_1+\omega_2) & 0 \\
0 & 0 & 0 & 0 & \alpha & 0 & 0 & 0
\end{pmatrix}.$$

Substituting the parameters value in Table 1, the eigenvalues of the matrix J_0 are $\lambda_1 = 1.110913, \lambda_2 = 0, \lambda_3 = -0.00669, \lambda_4 = -0.00670, \lambda_5 = -0.07066, \lambda_6 = -0.19944, \lambda_7 = -0.74398, \lambda_8 = -2.10655$. Since some eigenvalues are real positive and others are real negative, E_0 is unstable (van den Driessche and Watmough, 2002), indicating that the disease persist in the host population in the absence of preventive/curative measures and there is no need of analysing the endemic point. The implication of this is that preventive and control measures should be stepped up in order to control the spreading epidemic.

4.2.   Basic Reproduction Number

The concept of the basic reproduction number [4] is an important parameter in epidemiology that gives an indication of how much efforts are needed to control epidemics. If a prevention, intervention, or control strategy such as vaccination, social distancing, treatment is aimed at all individuals regardless of their epidemiological status, the value of the basic reproduction number is a measure of the strength of the control required to prevent outbreaks from occurring in a given population (Shuai et al., 2013).

Generally, to compute the basic reproduction number we follow the algorithm developed by van den Driessche and Watmough (2002). Let $X = (X_i, i = 1, 2, \ldots, n)$ denote the number or proportion of individuals in the ith compartment. Also, let $\mathscr{F}_i(X)$ be the rate of appearance of new infections in compartment i, and $\mathscr{V}_i = \mathscr{V}_i^- - \mathscr{V}_i^+$ be the rate of transfer of individuals into $(\mathscr{V}_i^+)$ and out $(\mathscr{V}_i^-)$ of compartment i. Note that each function $(\mathscr{F}_i(X), \mathscr{V}_i^+, \mathscr{V}_i^-)$ is assumed to be continuously differentiable at least twice with respect to each variable (Heffernan et al., 2005). The difference $\mathscr{F}_i(X) - \mathscr{V}_i(X)$ gives the rate of change in X. The basic reproduction number computed at the disease free equilibrium is the most dominant eigenvalue of the next generation matrix FV^{-1}. The new infections from all other changes in the population include: exposed, quarantine, isolated, infected and dead individuals.

$$\frac{dE(t)}{dt} = \frac{S(t)}{N}(\beta(t)I(t) + \rho D(t)) - (k + w + \mu)E(t),$$

$$\frac{dQ(t)}{dt} = wE(t) - (p_1 + p_2 + \mu)Q(t),$$

---

[4]The basic reproduction number is the average number of secondary infections generated by one infected individual of Ebola in a population where every individual is susceptible. It determines whether an infectious disease dies out or spreads in the population (van den Driessche and Watmough, 2002).

$$\frac{dI(t)}{dt} = kE(t) + p_2 Q(t) - (\gamma_1 + \gamma_2 + \gamma_3 + \mu)I(t),$$

$$\frac{dJ(t)}{dt} = \gamma_2 I(t) - (\omega_1 + \omega_2 + \mu)J(t), \tag{4}$$

$$\frac{dD(t)}{dt} = \gamma_3 I(t) + \omega_2 J(t) - \alpha D(t),$$

From the system (4), $\mathscr{F}$ and $\mathscr{V}$ are given respectively by :

$$\mathscr{F} = \begin{pmatrix} \beta I + \rho D \\ 0 \\ 0 \\ 0 \\ 0 \end{pmatrix}, \quad \text{and} \quad \mathscr{V} = \begin{pmatrix} (k+w+\mu)E \\ (p_1 + p_2 + \mu)Q \\ -kE - p_2 Q + (\gamma_1 + \gamma_2 + \gamma_3 + \mu)I \\ -\gamma_2 I + (\omega_1 + \omega_2 + \mu)J \\ -\gamma_3 I - \omega_2 J + \alpha D \end{pmatrix},$$

Given E_0 as the disease free equilibrium, we calculate the non-negative matrix F and the non-singular matrix V as follows. $F = \left[\frac{\partial \mathscr{F}_i(E_0)}{\partial X_j}\right]$ and $V = \left[\frac{\partial \mathscr{V}_i(E_0)}{\partial X_j}\right]$. i and j run from 1 to 5 denote the number of infected classes (Heffernan et al., 2005).

We therefore have;

$$F = \begin{pmatrix} 0 & 0 & \beta & 0 & \rho \\ 0 & 0 & 0 & 0 & 0 \\ 0 & 0 & 0 & 0 & 0 \\ 0 & 0 & 0 & 0 & 0 \\ 0 & 0 & 0 & 0 & 0 \end{pmatrix}, \text{and } V = \begin{pmatrix} k & 0 & 0 & 0 & 0 \\ 0 & p_2 & 0 & 0 & 0 \\ -k & -p_2 & \gamma_1 + \gamma_2 + \gamma_3 & 0 & 0 \\ 0 & 0 & -\gamma_2 & \omega_1 + \omega_2 & 0 \\ 0 & 0 & -\gamma_3 & -\omega_2 & \alpha \end{pmatrix},$$

The next generation matrix FV^{-1} is given by;

$$FV^{-1} = \begin{pmatrix} Z_1 + Z_2 & Z_3 + Z_4 & Z_5 & Z_6 & \frac{\rho}{\alpha} \\ 0 & 0 & 0 & 0 & 0 \\ 0 & 0 & 0 & 0 & 0 \\ 0 & 0 & 0 & 0 & 0 \\ 0 & 0 & 0 & 0 & 0 \end{pmatrix}, \tag{5}$$

where

$$Z_1 = \frac{\rho}{\alpha} \left(\frac{\gamma_3}{\gamma_1 + \gamma_2 + \gamma_3 + \mu} \left(\frac{k}{k + \mu + w} + \frac{p_2 w}{(k + \mu + w)(\mu + p_1 + p_2)} \right) + \eta \right);$$

$$Z_2 = \frac{\beta}{\gamma_1 + \gamma_2 + \gamma_3 + \mu} \left(\frac{k}{k + \mu + w} + \frac{p_2 w}{(k + \mu + w)(\mu + p_1 + p_2)} \right);$$

$$Z_3 = \frac{\rho}{\alpha} \left(\frac{\gamma_3 p_2}{(\gamma_1 + \gamma_2 + \gamma_3 + \mu)(\mu + p_1 + p_2)} + \frac{\gamma_2 \omega_2 p_2}{(\gamma_1 + \gamma_2 + \gamma_3 + \mu)(\mu + \omega_1 + \omega_2)(\mu + p_1 + p_2)} \right);$$

$$Z_4 = \frac{\beta p_2}{(\gamma_1 + \gamma_2 + \gamma_3 + \mu)(\mu + p_1 + p_2)};$$

$$Z_5 = \frac{\rho}{\alpha} \left(\frac{\gamma_3}{\gamma_1 + \gamma_2 + \gamma_3 + \mu} + \frac{\gamma_2 \omega_2}{(\gamma_1 + \gamma_2 + \gamma_3 + \mu)(\mu + \omega_1 + \omega_2)} \right) + \frac{\beta}{\gamma_1 + \gamma_2 + \gamma_3 + \mu};$$

$$Z_6 = \frac{\omega_2 \rho}{\alpha(\mu + \omega_1 + \omega_2)},$$

with

$$\eta = \frac{\gamma_2 \omega_2}{(\gamma_1 + \gamma_2 + \gamma_3 + \mu)(\mu + \omega_1 + \omega_2)} \left(\frac{k}{k + \mu + w} + \frac{p_2 w}{(k + \mu + w)(\mu + p_1 + p_2)} \right)$$

Since the matrix in (5) is an upper triangle matrix, the set of eigenvalues is the set of elements in the main diagonal, that is $\{(Z_1 + Z_2, 0, 0, 0, 0)\}$.

Therefore, the dominant eigenvalue (R_0) of the obtained next generation matrix is given by;

$$R_0 = Z_1 + Z_2. \tag{6}$$

By substituting the estimated values from Table 1 in (6), we obtain $R_0 = 2.79$. That is, on average, one infected individual can infect 3 individuals in the whole susceptible population during his entire period of infectiousness. The closest value in the literature to our estimate is $R_0 = 2.7$ by Legrand et al. (2007). A summary of various reproduction numbers of Ebola models can be found in (Barbarossa et al., 2015; Shen et al., 2015).

5. Numerical Simulations

5.1. Model Solution

In order to investigate what effect do isolation and quarantine have on the number of Ebola cases and deaths, we carry out numerical simulations of the model

1. Given our model parameter values, we graphically examine the long term dynamic of quarantine and isolation (see Figure 2a). The model is then fitted to daily data and one notes that the synthetic data fit the model almost perfectly, (see Figure 2b).

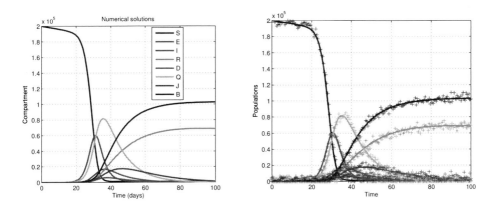

Figure 2. Ebola epidemic model numerical simulations.

The susceptible variable is decreasing since some of its candidates are immigrating to E. By this time, E, Q, I, J and D are increasing and decrease after a certain period. R and B are increasing exponentially. The model numerical solutions are also fitted to simulated daily data. With synthetic data, it is evident that the model clearly fits the daily data.

Even if the model fits the generated data, the coefficient of determination is computed to ascertain the level as below

$$R^2 = 1 - \frac{\sum (Y_i - f(Y_i, \hat{\theta}))^2}{\sum (Y_i - \bar{Y}_i)^2},$$

where $\hat{\theta}$ and $\bar{Y}_i$ are estimated parameters and mean of data respectively.

5.2. Parameters Identification Using MCMC Method

In MCMC method, the parameter of interest is assigned a prior distribution $\theta \sim \pi(\bullet)$. In this Bayesian inference, the goal is to estimate the chain of posteriors θ given the data y, which is obtained via the Bayes formula $p(\theta \mid y) \propto$

$f(y; \theta)\pi(\theta)$. We then obtain the estimators of θ by considering the posterior mean $\mathbb{E}[\theta, y]$ or the median of the posterior distribution, for instance (Ndanguza, 2015; Ndanguza et al., 2016). Posterior distribution is defined as the conditional probability distribution of some parameter with respect to some observed data. The mean and median of the posterior distribution are respectively referred to as posterior mean and posterior median.

We use the Metropolis-Hastings algorithm (Ndanguza, 2015) with 100,000 number of simulations to compute the chain of posteriors. It is described as below

---

Algorithm 1 Metropolis-Hastings algorithm

---

1. start with an arbitrary value θ_0,

2. update from θ_n to $\theta_{n+1} (n = 0, 1, \ldots)$ by

   - generate $\xi \sim q(\xi | \theta_n)$,
   - evaluate $\alpha(\theta_n, \xi) = \min\left(1, \frac{\pi(\xi)q(\xi, \theta_n)}{\pi(\theta_n)q(\theta_n, \xi)}\right)$,
   - set
   $$\theta_{n+1} = \begin{cases} \xi & \text{with probability } \alpha, \\ \theta_n & \text{otherwise.} \end{cases}$$

The distribution $\pi(\theta)$ is often called the *target* distribution whereas the distribution with density $q(.|\theta)$ is the *proposal* distribution. For more MCMC algorithms refer to (Brooks, 1998; Geyer, 1992; Tierney, 1994; Brooks and Roberts, 1998; Ndanguza, 2015; Ndanguza et al., 2016) among others. Table 2 compares the estimates from LSQ methods and posteriors mean.

Plotting and inspecting traces and histograms of the observed MCMC sample is the most straightforward approach for assessing chains' convergence to the stationary distribution, which is also our target distribution. MCMC algorithms create a sample from the posterior distribution, and we inspect whether this sample is sufficiently close to the posterior to be used for analysis (Ndanguza, 2015). However, there is a doubt of ascertaining whether our chain will normally converge after K draws. Since no one can not be sure, there are several tests which can be used, both visual and statistical, to see if the chain appears to

Table 2. Comparison of the estimated model parameters using synthetic data by LSQ and MCMC methods

Parameters	Initial values	LSQ	Posterior mean	Posterior median	Posterior std
β_0	8.2624	8.2953	8.1910	8.1415	0.7101
β_1	0.0187	0.0188	17.9241	7.4348	34.5777
$1/k$	3.248	3.2419	3.3078	3.2858	0.2161
$1/\gamma_1$	8.2281	8.2925	10.7415	10.6833	1.0015
$1/\gamma_2$	8.1921	8.2562	8.4600	8.4369	0.7771
$1/\gamma_3$	3.6946	3.7235	3.8690	3.8652	0.2854
ω_1	0.0521	0.0525	0.0143	0.0143	0.0024
ω_2	0.0112	0.0113	0.0097	0.0097	0.0025
p_1	0.0107	0.0106	0.0177	0.0173	0.0062
p_2	0.0938	0.0945	0.0937	0.0937	0.0033
w	0.2707	0.2728	0.2838	0.2832	0.0144
α	0.7593	0.7225	0.9539	0.8974	0.2612

have converged.

Among those tests, graphical display is an important component of the MCMC method (Ndanguza et al., 2017). It provides the visual displays of MCMC output for checking the behavior from the random sampling process, including convergence of Markov chains and independency of samples (Ndanguza, 2015).

One of the methods for checking lack of convergence is to visualize the scatter plots of several MCMC chains initialized with different starting values (Tierney, 1994). Below in Figure 3, we test the convergence using the MCMC trace plot and Marginal density plot. Figure 3 indicates that mixing of the samples is relatively good except for the parameter β_1 where the trace plot does not show a stationarity and the marginal density plot is not normal as it should. Since this parameter β_1 is the contact rate after the outbreak, this lack of normality is due to the uncertainty encountered in predicting when the outbreak will die out. Hence, there is a high variance in the chain.

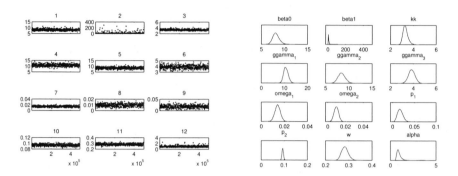

Figure 3. The model MCMC trace plot and Marginal density plot.

Conclusion

Ebola is a rare and deadly disease transmissible disease which has been resurgent in recent years (2014 West Africa outbreak). We formulated a mathematical model of the transmission dynamic of the disease, considering vital dynamics and two non-therapeutic intervention measures: isolation and quarantine. These prevention strategies were implemented during the 2014 West Africa Ebola outbreak. The proposed model is a refinement of the model proposed by Ndanguza et al. (2013). MCMC algorithm and LSQ methods are used to estimate the model parameters. Furthermore, to reduce the simulation uncertainties, the unknown model parameters were identified by the MCMC technique and Least Square methods in order to generate reasonable model parameter estimates. The model basic reproduction number R_0 which represents the number of secondary cases generated by an index case in the absence of any control measure was calculated both analytically and numerically. The value of $R_0 = 2.79$ is slightly higher than the values computed in other Ebola epidemics/models (see Shen et al. (2015)), with often slightly different set of parameter values (Chowell et al., 2004; Chowell and Nishiura, 2014; Ndanguza et al., 2013) indicates that on average, one infected individual could have potentially infected 3 susceptible individuals, and this could explain the magnitude and severity of the 2014 epidemic in the region. The long-term dynamics of the model was investigated numerically. Finally, the model was then fitted to daily synthetic data and it was observed that the model fits the data at 96%.

Conflict of Interest

The authors declare that there is no conflict of interest regarding the publication of this paper.

References

Agusto, F. B., Teboh-Ewungkem, M. I., and Gumel, A. B. (2015). Mathematical assessment of the effect of traditional beliefs and customs on the transmission dynamics of the 2014 Ebola outbreaks. *BMC Medicine*, 13(1):96.

Banton, S., Roth, Z., and Pavlovic, M. (2010). Mathematical modeling of Ebola virus dynamics as a step towards rational vaccine design. *26th Southern Biomedical Engineering Conference SBEC, April 30 - May 2, 2010, College Park, Maryland, USA IFMBE Proceedings*, 32:196-200.

Barbarossa, M. V., Dénes, A., Kiss, G., Nakata, Y., Röst, G., and Vizi, Z. (2015). Transmission dynamics and final epidemic size of Ebola virus disease outbreaks with varying interventions. *PloS ONE*, 10(7):e0131398.

Bashar, S., Percy, M., and Singhai, R. (2014). *Predicting the 2014 Ebola outbreak in West Africa using network analysis.* http://snap.stanford.edu/class/cs224w-2014/projects2014/cs224w-45-final.pdf. Accessed 30th June, 2017.

Berge, T., Lubuma, J.-S., Moremedi, G., Morris, N., and Kondera-Shava, R. (2017). A simple mathematical model for Ebola in Africa. *Journal of Biological Dynamics*, 11(1):42–74.

Brooks, S. (1998). Markov chain Monte Carlo method and its application. *Journal of the Royal Statistical Society: Series D (the Statistician)*, 47(1):69–100.

Brooks, S. P. and Roberts, G. O. (1998). Assessing convergence of Markov chain Monte Carlo algorithms. *Statistics and Computing*, 8(4):319–335.

Camacho, A., Kucharski, A., Funk, S., Breman, J., Piot, P., and Edmunds, W. (2014). Potential for large outbreaks of Ebola virus disease. *Epidemics*, 9:70–78.

CDC (2016). *Ebola virus disease.* http://www.cdc.gov/vhf/ebola/about.html. Accessed on 4th June, 2016.

Chowell, G., Hengartner, N., Castillo-Chavez, C., and Hyman, P. F. J. (2004). The basic reproductive number of Ebola and the effects of public health measures: the case of Congo and Uganda. *Journal of Theoretical Biology*, 229(E2):119-126.

Chowell, G. and Nishiura, H. (2014). Transmission dynamics and control of Ebola virus disease (EVD): a review. *BMC Medicine*, 12(1):196.

Demiris, N. (2004). *Bayesian Inference for stochastic epidemic models using Markov chain Monte Carlo Methods.* PhD thesis, University of Nottingham.

Downing, D. J., Gardner, R., and Hoffman, F. (1985). An examination of response-surface methodologies for uncertainty analysis in assessment models. *Technometrics*, 27(2):151–163.

Geyer, C. J. (1992). Practical Markov chain Monte Carlo. *Statistical Science*, pages 473–483.

Hamby, D. (1994). A review of techniques for parameter sensitivity analysis of environmental models. *Environmental Monitoring and Assessment*, 32(2):135–154.

Heffernan, J., Smith, R., and Wahl, L. (2005). Perspectives on the basic reproductive ratio. *Journal of the Royal Society Interface*, 2(4):281–293.

Hethcote, H. (2000). The mathematics of infectious diseases. *SIAM Review*, 42:599-653.

Hethcote, H., Zhien, M., and Shengbing, L. (2002). Effects of quarantine in six endemic models for infectious diseases. *Mathematical Biosciences*, 180(E2):141-160.

Khan, A., Naveed, M., Dur-e Ahmad, M., and Imran, M. (2015). Estimating the basic reproductive ratio for the Ebola outbreak in Liberia and Sierra Leone. *Infectious Diseases of Poverty*, 4(1):13.

Legrand, J., Grais, R., Boelle, P., Valleron, A., and Flahault, A. (2007). Understanding the dynamics of Ebola epidemics. *Epidemiology and Infection*, 135(04):610–621.

Lekone, P. and Finkenstadt, B. (2006). Statistical inference in a stochastic epidemic SEIR model with control intervention: Ebola as a case study. *Biometrics*, 62:1170-1177.

Lewnard, J. A., Mbah, M. L. N., Alfaro-Murillo, J. A., Altice, F. L., Bawo, L., Nyenswah, T. G., and Galvani, A. P. (2014). Dynamics and control of Ebola virus transmission in Montserrado, Liberia: a mathematical modelling analysis. *The Lancet Infectious Diseases*, 14(12):1189–1195.

Morgan, B. J. T. (2000). *Applied Stochastic modelling*. Oxford University Press Inc.

Ndanguza, D., Mbalawata, I., and Nsabimana, J. (2016). Analysis of SDEs applied to SEIR epidemic models by extended Kalman filter method. *Applied Mathematics*, 7(17):2195–2211.

Ndanguza, D., Mbalawata, I. S., Haario, H., and Tchuenche, J. M. (2017). Analysis of bias in an Ebola epidemic model by extended Kalman filter approach. *Mathematics and Computers in Simulation*, 142:113–129.

Ndanguza, D., Tchuenche, J., and Haario, H. (2013). Statistical data analysis of the 1995 Ebola outbreak in the Democratic Republic of Congo. *Afrika Matematika*, 24(1):55-68.

Ndanguza, R. D. (2015). Bayesian analysis of SEIR epidemic models. *Acta Universitatis Lappeenrantaensis*.

Newman, M. E. (2002). Spread of epidemic disease on networks. *Physical Review E*, 66(1):016128.

Rivers, C., Lofgren, E., Marathe, M., Eubank, S., and BL, L. (2014). Modeling the impact of interventions on an epidemic of Ebola in Sierra Leone and Liberia. *PLOS Currents Outbreaks*.

Robert, P. and Casella, G. (2004). *Monte Carlo Statistical Methods*. New York, USA: Springer-Verlag.

Salaam-Blyther, T. (2014). The 2014 Ebola outbreak: International and US responses. *Current Politics and Economics of Africa*, 7(4):523.

Shen, M., Xiao, Y., and Rong, L. (2015). Modeling the effect of comprehensive interventions on ebola virus transmission. *Scientific reports*, 5:15818.

Shuai, Z., Heesterbeek, J., and van den Driessche, P. (2013). Extending the type reproduction number to infectious disease control targeting contacts between types. *Journal of Mathematical Biology*, 67(5):1067–1082.

Tierney, L. (1994). Markov chains for exploring posterior distributions. *The Annals of Statistics*, pages 1701–1728.

van den Driessche, P. and Watmough, J. (2002). Reproduction numbers and sub-threshold endemic equilibria for compartmental models of disease transmission. *Mathematical Biosciences*, 180(1):29–48.

Webb, G. and Browne, C. (2016). A model of the Ebola epidemics in West Africa incorporating age of infection. *Journal of Biological Dynamics*, 10(1):18–30.

Yamin, D., Gertler, S., Ndeffo-Mbah, M. L., Skrip, L. A., Fallah, M., Nyenswah, T. G., Altice, F. L., and Galvani, A. P. (2015). Effect of ebola progression on transmission and control in liberia. *Annals of internal medicine*, 162(1):11–17.

Yi, N., Zhang, Q., Mao, K., Yang, D., , and Li, Q. (2009). Analysis and control of an SEIR epidemic system with nonlinear transmission rate. *Mathematical and Computer Modelling*, 50:1498-1513.

In: Ebola Virus Disease (EVD)   ISBN: 978-1-53616-291-2
Editor: Hilaire Verreau   © 2019 Nova Science Publishers, Inc.

Chapter 2

PREVENTIVE AND CONTROL MEASURES OF EBOLA VIRAL DISEASE OUTBREAK: A RACE AGAINST TIME AND CULTURAL PRACTICES

Chidiebere E. Ugwu[1,], Ernest Tambo[2,3] and Stephen M. Suru[1]*

[1]Department of Human Biochemistry,
Faculty of Basic Medical Sciences,
Nnamdi Azikiwe University Nnewi Campus,
Nnewi, Anambra State Nigeria
[2]Higher Institute of Health Sciences, Universite des Mointagnes,
Banagangte, Cameroon
[3]Africa intelligence and communications, Yaounde, Cameroon

---

* Corresponding Author's Email: Ce.ugwu@unizik.edu.ng; ugwuchidiksu@yahoo.com.

ABSTRACT

At present, there is no vaccine against Ebola Virus suggesting a stalemate in man's effort to curb this extremely fatal disease. This life-threatening scenario implies that prevention and control measure of Ebola Virus Disease (EVD) are predominantly centered on case identification and isolation, early broad-based medical care, surveillance of suspected cases, and safe burial practices. Optimizing the existing control and prevention strategies such as community engagement and awareness, improved access to personal protective equipment (PPE), Community Care Centers (CCC) and EVD treatment (if any) are pivotal in the prevention and control strategy. The preliminary key to a successful outbreak control is hinged on community engagement by creating awareness to risk factors and prevention measures. The importance of vaccine to combat the disease is also highlighted. The chapter also discussed humanitarian issues in EVD prevention and control and humanitarian protection during EVD outbreak and the challenges posed by cultural practices and social norms during outbreaks. Some innovative approaches in the humanitarian response to prevention and control have been discussed.

Keywords: Ebola, outbreaks, humanitarian emergency, prevention, control.

INTRODUCTION

The Ebola Virus Disease (EVD) is an extremely contagious, fatal and untreatable disease in man and nonhuman primates. Initial symptoms range from sudden fever, intense weakness, muscle pain and sore throat to severe symptoms of vomiting, diarrhea, internal and external bleeding, culminating in death. The disease is transmitted to humans through close contact with infected animals, including chimpanzees, fruit bats and forest antelope. The African fruit bats of the family *Pteropodidae* are taught to be the reservoir host (Goldstein et al., 2018). Contact with infected living or dead animal is the major mode of transmission to humans and is spread in human population by human-to-human close physical contact with infected blood, bodily fluids or organs, or indirectly through contact with contaminated environments (Ngatu et al., 2017). Even funerals of Ebola victims can be a risk, if mourners have direct contact with the body of the deceased. Healthcare workers are at risk if they treat patients without taking the right precautions to avoid infection. People are infectious as long as their blood and secretions contain the virus - in some cases, up to seven weeks after they recover. The incubation period is two days to three weeks, and diagnosis is difficult.

The Ebola Virus Disease was first discovered in the Democratic Republic of Congo in 1976 and since then it has affected countries further east, including Uganda and Sudan. The recent outbreak in West Africa is unusual and unprecedented because of the fact that the cases were scattered in multiple locations that has never before been affected, rapid spread to other countries, highest mortality rate and with the deadliest and most aggressive strain of the virus (Baseler et al., 2017). The 2014-2016 EVD outbreak in five West African Countries outnumbered all previous Ebola outbreaks in the number of confirmed cases and mortality which made the World Health Organization (WHO) to declare a Public Health Emergency of International Concern (PHEIC) (Shears and O'Dempsey, 2015). Since its emergence in 1976, understanding the pathways of transmission has reduced the mortality rate of the disease outbreaks. The human disease has so far been mostly limited to Africa, although one strain has cropped up in the Philippines.

OPTIMIZING EBOLA OUTBREAK COMMUNITY-BASED PREVENTION AND CONTROL STRATEGIES

A positive outbreak control depends on applying a feasible intervention packages such as case management, surveillance and response system, contact tracing, adequate laboratory testing, community engagement, safe burial practices and social mobilization. The key to a successful outbreak control is community engagement by creating awareness to the risk factors and preventive measures (RCCE, 2018).

Community based methods to prevention and care could reduce Ebola infection (Pronyk et al., 2016). Also community engagement can enhance awareness and shift standards around major risk behavior (Rosaro et al., 2008). Engaging community and local leaders including religious and institutional leaders should be an effective control measure of the virus. They should be an integral part of the community engagement and awareness to create trust and security. Conflicts that will arise between key infection control measures and current cultural and traditional norms shall be better resolved internally.

There should be participatory measures to encourage prevention, quick referral and safe burials in alliance with community influencers and youth groups to actively involve community members in the development of their home grown response plans (Meredith et al., 2015). The outbreak response team should listen to the communities by engaging community influencers and responding to their community needs thereby adopting their interventions and services appropriately (Tambo et al., 2014; 2017).

The communities must be integrated in the planning and setting up of the disease containment centres which are necessary for early referral. Community engagement, improving the capacity of affected communities to prevent and control Ebola outbreak, is vital to nurturing trust and confidence in outbreak control pathways and inadvertently to break the mode of transmission (UNMEER, 2015). Active community engagement will improve people confidence in making early case referrals. The international outbreak response groups must provide communication skills to community influencers to increase their confidence level in effectively communicating with their people. Active case discovery can only be feasible if trust has been established between the response groups, community health volunteers and families. The families must be strengthened on basic case findings to guarantee effective referral of likely Ebola case (Meredith et al., 2015).

IMPROVED ACCESS TO PERSONAL PROTECTIVE EQUIPMENT (PPE)

The probability of transmission of Ebola virus can be limited if correct measures are applied especially in the use of Personal Protective Equipment (PPE). The transmission dynamics of the virus demands an immediate need for PPE due to lessons learnt from the 2014-2016 unprecedented EVD outbreak in West Africa (WHO, 2016; Reidy et al., 2017). While PPE is the most visible control used to prevent transmission, it must be used in conjunction with administration and engineering controls (WHO, 2016).

The inappropriate use or lack of PPE is one of the serious gaps in implementing infection and control standards in communities where transmission probably took place or where infected Health Care Workers (HCW) were employed (Reidy et al., 2017). There are evidences from the field that HCWs lack basic skills in the removal of PPE which led to contamination and endangered the HCWs (Casanova et al., 2016; Tomas et al., 2015). The quality of the PPE ought to be monitored and observed failures lodged through a formal reporting process. The criteria for selecting PPE should include accessibility in different sizes, resilient to heat, sweat, and chemicals, least loss of dexterity, and marginal loss of movement (Reidy et al., 2017).

HCWs empowerment and training is paramount and should be provided in a graded manner to enable them implement best practice and safety measures at all levels (Gibson et al., 2016). At regular intervals refresher training is necessary for the HCWs to remind, update their knowledge and boost their confidence and competence with the PPE protocols (Reidy et al., 2017). It is the responsibility of the end-user to select appropriate PPE after a critical hazard assessment of the task involved and the environment. The end-user must ensure that the selected PPE meets the official government standards and that people are adequately trained in the use and disposal of PPE to prevent contamination

(CDC, 2018). The health authority should ensure that there is adequate and accessible stockpile of PPE during outbreaks.

VALUE OF STRENGTHENING EBOLA TREATMENT AND COMMUNITY CARE CENTRES

The Ebola Treatment Centre (ETC) is a basic and pragmatic place for managing Ebola cases with high degree of infection prevention and control practice (Olu et al., 2015). They are settings used for isolating patients and providing clinical care. Typically, such centre should have large capacity and operate under high level of infection control (Kucharski et al., 2015). The basic aspect of ETCs is stratifying those infected according to their individual likelihood of having the disease thereby decreasing the risk of having nosocomial Ebola infection within the facility (Janke et al., 2017).

At present, the one of the major setback with the Ebola treatment unit is that it is less effective in managing the needs of non-Ebola patients as it lacks differential therapeutic routines for non-Ebola conditions (Janke et al., 2017). With the unprecedented experience of 2014-2015 Ebola crises in Sierra Leone and Liberia, the ETCs reaching capacity patients were overwhelmed. In the situation were the ETC capacity is out stripped with patients, many suspected or probable cases would remain in their respective homes thereby increasing the likelihood of secondary infection of family members and community transmission of the virus (Whitty et al., 2014). This scenario may necessitate the urgent need to rapidly scale up treatment and isolation facilities. Hence, the need for Community Care Centres (CCC) to support the ETCs.

The ETCs are complex setup that requires a good number of staff and time to start up. In view of this, the WHO and other response organizations considered CCC as the next care option to complement and augment the ETCs (Kuchaski et al., 2015). The CCC plays a complimentary role to conventional ETCs. It enhances the capacity for early case detection and improves access to Ebola Care at community mobilization, participation in safe and decent burial (Pronyk et al., 2016). The CCC should be an adjunct in the management of EVD cases during outbreaks (Olu et al., 2015). The CCC can complement the ETC thus:

- It will promote better community mobilization and ownership of the outbreak response efforts thereby enhancing early identification and isolation of cases at the rural level.
- Community engagement in the process shall provide avenue for mobilization into action.
- The CCC will reduce the pressure on the district hospitals to concentrate on providing basic primary health care.

EBOLA IMMUNIZATION PROGRAMS AND OTHER PROTECTIVE STRATEGIES

The fast progression of the virus that does not allow for the development of natural immunity shows that vaccination may be a promising intervention to stop infection and limit spread. The 2014 outbreak of EVD brought to light the immediate need for a licensed vaccine to curb future outbreaks of the disease and has significantly accelerated vaccine development with many candidate vaccines already at clinical phases (Sridher, 2015; Gross et al., 2018; Venkartraman et al., 2018). Our findings showed that 36 trials of Ebola vaccine candidates have been completed and another 14 are active, according to clinicaltrials.gov. The humanitarian community should be quickly mobilized to launch significant coordination and advocacy initiatives.

It is impossible to evaluate clinical protection from the virus in human population outside epidemic period while in non-epidemic situation; the antibody response following vaccination with Ebola candidate vaccines is the criterion presently in use for evaluation. Results from clinical trials indicate high level of uncertainty in the determinants of antibody response as a result of preventive vaccination against EVD (Gross et al., 2018). For preventive purpose, vaccination of health care workers has substantial potential of minimizing scale and duration of outbreaks (WHO/SAGE, 2018).

Overall, the major task facing the global health community is to ensure that in future outbreaks there is a licensed vaccine to combat at least two major virulent strains of the Ebola virus isolated in human infections (Sullivan et al., 2000). The longevity of protection, best deployment approaches and mechanistic immunological correlates are some of the many unanswered questions toward the licensing of a new vaccine against the Ebola virus. (Venkartraman et al., 2018). Also protection in specific human sub groups such as children and pregnant women remains to be addressed (Gross et al., 2018).

In order to achieve success in spite of these challenges, emphasis should be on intensive and sustained Ebola vaccination communication and community engagement strategies in conflict and remote rural communities coupled with the community-based emergency preparedness and rapid response programs. The treatments can be used as long as informed consent is obtained from patients and protocols are followed, with close monitoring and reporting of any adverse events, under the framework of compassionate use/expanded access. Affected countries should be supported in establishing ETCs and providing clinical care, partners and experts consultation in the field of Ebola vaccination and drugs randomized controlled trials (RCTs) in affected conflict settings. Scientific communities and affected countries must collaborate with each other to collect and accumulate robust evidence over a number of outbreaks over a period of time and to refrain from seeing each outbreak as a discrete episode. These are crucial in increasing community health promotion and community mobilization, resilience and relief access and utilization including the use of investigational therapeutics or investigational vaccine(s) for post-exposure prophylaxis (PEP) for frontline healthcare workers (HCWs) potentially exposed to Ebola virus (Zaire ebolavirus) during outbreaks. Sequel to this, national immunization schedules and regional mass immunization programs should be scaled up to help the communities (Tambo et al., 2015).

HUMANITARIAN ETHICAL, CULTURAL AND LEGAL ISSUES AND CHALLENGES IN EBOLA OUTBREAK EMERGENCY RESPONSE

The outbreak of Ebola virus disease unveiled the main weaknesses and ineffectiveness in the global humanitarian health management and prompted the emergence of new and more robust methods of responding to the crisis by modifying how we organize humanitarian and civil protection resources jointly (Florika-Hooijer, 2015). The West Africa Ebola crisis got out of control because the humanitarian global clusters relevant to Ebola response were not mobilized on time to support the impoverished local capacity (Perache, 2015).

The global response system to such crisis has to be reviewed for synergy in the leadership and coordination of International humanitarian agency and international health control. It is apparent from recent outbreak that the activities of the local-based humanitarian bodies are not efficiently governed to make a quick request for global support. More so, the national governments of countries affected should be transparent in information management to create proper response and quick engagement of Global Health Cluster resources. Resident coordinators of major global health players including the WHO are to be properly equipped and aware of the resources available for emergencies. For effective humanitarian response, the Health Clusters should be mobilized early whenever it becomes clear that needs are increasing more than the capacity of response.

Furthermore, there should be a coordinated early deployment of foreign medical groups to help solve problems of low-key operation capacity. An early request by the national government for international assistance will create avenue for quick response to support the week health system on ground. The frontline issues in humanitarian response can be addressed by providing health and humanitarian personnel and equipment early. The safety of the personnel must be guaranteed by the host community before deployment of the experts. This underscores the need for rapid and continued humanitarian and peace building efforts to develop an effective and lasting solutions and livelihoods.

REINFORCING HUMANITARIAN PROTECTION DURING EBOLA OUTBREAK EMERGENCY CRISIS

How do we protect the vulnerable from abuse during crisis such as Ebola outbreak? It is generally agreed that humanitarian emergencies irrespective of cause, reproduces fresh vulnerabilities. These emergencies place the vulnerable groups to heightened risk and destroy traditional and social systems that control behavior. There is increased chance of gender-based violence including girl-child sex abuse (Kahn, 2015).

Women and children must be given attention during humanitarian crisis such as Ebola in order not to exacerbate the existing vulnerabilities they face. Children separated from their families due to Ebola crisis should be systematically identified and reunited with their families or placed with a care giver and their well-being followed up. Specific protection and assistance to child or female should be adequately provided to reduce abuse. The most vulnerable groups must be protected by accommodating them in the disease prevention and protection strategy by dedicating specific transportation, isolation and treatment services to them. There should be specific facilities to care for pregnant women, children without families and people with disabilities. The dignity of the vulnerable groups should be upheld while children should be separated from adults and men and from women where facilities exist. The humanitarian groups and care givers in the treatment facilities should not abuse survivors undergoing convalescence. Stigmatization surrounding Ebola is one of the greatest challenges health workers face.

The humanitarian response to protection during Ebola crisis should be led by personnel that understand protection from humanitarian perspective and not a public health approach. All humanitarian response should have dignity and humanity of the affected communities at the centre of the response. The focus on humanitarian and public health aspect of the response must be synergized to achieve the objective of zero cases. A major lesson learnt in the 2014-2016 West Africa Ebola outbreak was the importance of providing funds and resources early for protection activities. There should be methods to fast-track reconciliation and reintegration to those that survives Ebola and abuses that follow such outbreaks.

RACE AGAINST TIME AND CULTURAL PRACTICES

Ebola Virus Disease is extremely contagious and strikes with a lightning speed. Comparatively, the so-called 'rapid' response and implementation of control measures are often of the speed of snail. Beyond existing weak health system and surveillance, movement of people, especially those infected, is very difficult to control. In some cases, infected people are defiant of restriction of movement order as in the case of infected Dr Samuel Brisbane, who left Liberia for Nigeria. Out of mistaken love or fear of dying alone, some people deliberately ignore restriction order and visit sick people or uninfected relatives without any protective equipment. Also, some infected people are not aware of their being infected, such that they continue on their daily routine thereby risking infecting others.

Ebola outbreaks occur primarily in remote villages in Central and West Africa, near tropical rainforests were adherence to cultural practices are predominant and insufficient levels of access to uptake of lifesaving medical care and prevention strategies exist. Cultural practices around religion and death involve close physical contact among mourners, undertakers and the dead. Hugging is a normal part of religious worship and across the region the ritual preparation of bodies for burial involves washing, touching and kissing. Those with the highest status or certain age group grade in society are often charged with washing and preparing the body. For a woman this can include braiding the hair, and for a man shaving the head and manicure. Strongly entrenched is the transportation and burial of corpse at home town of the deceased. Fatal victims of Ebola usually have a very high viral load of the virus and those who handle the body and come into contact with the blood or other body fluids are at greatest risk of being infected and/or serve as heavy carrier of the virus.

More so, consumption of bush meat has long been part of the people. Fruit bats, monkeys, apes and African rabbits in particular are considered delicacies in these areas of outbreak. Likewise, picking of falling fruits as freebies for consumption are not uncommon.

The aforementioned are part of the problems for many in the Central and West African countries usually affected by the outbreak. These therefore underscore the need to make people aware of how their treatment of dead relatives and unwholesome consumption of bush meat might pose a risk to themselves. This message, among others, has proved very difficult to pass across because such cultural treatments of the dead are cherished as heritage and viewed as honorable and sign of last respect.

EDUCATION/FEAR FACTOR

In places with previous outbreaks, the education message about avoiding contact has had years to enter the individual and collective consciousness of all. Sadly for some in West Africa, there simply has not been the time for the necessary cultural/social shift. At the initial stage of the outbreak in Nigeria, that perspective only changed theoretically as some view the Ebola outbreak as a conspiracy theory to deprive them of their supposed cultural heritage. Not left out are some of the citizens of the DR Congo who believed that Ebola was a hoax and a tactic used by the government to 'take the blood of the people', thus the resistance. But as death toll rises, especially among medical personnel, it became evident that this was not a conspiracy theory or hoax; the Ebola shroud has become an inevitable and horrendous reality.

The Ebola outbreak triggers fear because many have not experienced and/or forgotten what it is like to face something that strike with lightning speed and fatality rate. This scenario caused an unparalleled, momentous shift in social behavior and attitude: limited daily talking, public hand washing, use of sanitizers and increased daily salt use (drinking/bath) became the norms; handshake, touching/sitting where others previously had contacts, collection of cash balance after monetary transaction were frightening and uncanny etc. These scenarios were greeted with sad consequences; confusion, salt intoxication, increased blood pressure just to mention a few.

CONCLUSION

To truly conquer EVD, we need a comprehensive approach towards building on the meager success achieved in controlling and preventing Ebola outbreak in recent past. The need to double down on Ebola disease and make good use of the experiences and lessons to significantly avert outbreak is ever more critical. The need to invest in robust health systems that prioritize surveillance and rapid response services for combating Ebola disease is obligatory. The need for confirmed Ebola vaccine is indispensable and behind schedule. The need to renounce cultural practices that are capable of eliciting Ebola outbreak and/or detrimental to its control and preventive measures is non-negotiable. A constant public awareness campaigns on Ebola need stepped up. Campaigns will help communities to understand how much of a risk Ebola is, not only to neighboring countries but also to communities and global community during Ebola outbreaks.

REFERENCES

Baseler L, Chertow D, Johnson KM, Feldmann H, Morens DM. (2017). The pathogenesis of Ebola virus disease. *Annual Review of Pathology: Mechanisms of Disease*. 12:387-418.

Casanova LM, Teal LJ, Sickbert-Bennett EE, Anderson DJ, Sexton DJ, Rutala WA, Weber DJ, and CDC Prevention epicenters Program. (2016). Assessment of self-contamination during removal of personal protective equipment for Ebola patient care. *Infection Control and Hospital Epidemiology*. 37: 1156-61.

Center for Disease Control and Prevention. (2018).Question and Answers on Ebola. CDC.gov.http://www.cdc.gov/vhf/ebola/pdf/ebola.ga.pdf.

FLORIKA-Hooijer F. (2015). Civil protection and humanitarian aid in the Ebola response: lessons for the humanitarian system from the EU experience. *Humanitarian Exchange*. 64:3-5.

Gibson C, Fletcher T, Clay K, Griffiths A. (2016). Foreign medical outbreak: a UK military model of pre-deployment training and assurance. *Journal of the Royal Army Medical Corps*. 162:163-168.

Goldstein S J, Gbakima AA, Bird BH, Bangura J, Tremeau-Bravard A, Belaganahalli MN, Wells HL, Dhanota JK, Liang E, Grodus M, Jangra RK, DeJesus VA, Lasso G, Smith BR, Jambai A, Kamara BO, Kamara S, Bangura W, Monagin C, Shapira S, Johnson CK, Saylors K, Rubin EM, Chandran K, Ian Lipkin W and Mazet JAK. (2018). The discovery of *Bombali* virus adds further support for bats as hosts of Ebola viruses. *Nature Microbiology*. 3:1084-1089.

Gross L, Lhomme E, Pasin C, Richert L, Thiebaut R. (2018). Ebola vaccine development: systematic review of pre-clinical and clinical studies, and meta-analysis of determinants of antibody response variability after vaccination. *International Journal of Infectious Diseases*. 74: 83-96.

Janke C, Heim KM, Steinner F, Massaquol M, Gbanya MZ, Frey C and Froeschl G. (2017). Beyond Ebola treatment units: severe infection temporary treatment units as an essential element of Ebola case management during an outbreak. *BMC Infectious Diseases*. 17:124. doi 10.1186/s12879-017-2235-x.

Kahn C. (2015). Ebola and humanitarian protection. *Humanitarian Exchange;* 64:10-12.

Kucharski AJ, Camacho A, Checchi F, Waldman R, Grais RF, Cabnol J, Briand S, Baguelin M, Flasche S, Funk S, Edmunds WJ. (2015). Evaluation of the benefits and risks of introducing Ebola Community Care Centers in Sierra Leone. *Emerging Infectious Diseases*. 21(3)393-399.

Meredith C, Asibal M, WiederbergerAse, We M, Carter S. a bottom-up approach to the Ebola response. *Humanitarian Exchange*. 64, 2015; 15-17. Fenton W and Foley M (Editors).

Ngatu NR, Ksyembe NJ, Phillips EK, Okech-Ojony J, Patou-Musumari M, Gaspard-Kibukusa M, Madone-Mandina N, Godefroid-Mayala M, Mutaawe L, Manzengo C, Roger-Wumba D, Nojima S. 2017. Epidemiology of Ebola virus disease (EVD) and occupational EVD in health care workers in Sub-Saharan Africa: need for strengthened public health preparedness. *Journal of Epidemiology*. 27:455-461.

Olu O, Cormican M, Kamara K and Butt W. (2015). Community Care Center (CCC) as adjunct in the management of Ebola Virus Disease (EVD) cases during outbreaks: experience from Sierra Leone. *Pan African Medical Journal*. 22(sup.1):14.

Perache AH. (2015). 'To put out this fire, we must run into the burning building': a review of MSF's call for biological containment teams in West Africa. *Humanitarian Exchange*. 64: 5-7.

Pronyk P, Rogers B, Lee S, Bhatnagar A, Wolman Y, Monasch R, Hipgrave D, Salama P, Kucharski A, Chopra M, on behalf of UNICEF Sierra Leone Ebola Response Team. 2016. The effect of community-based prevention and care on Ebola transmission in Sierra Leone. *American Journal of Public Health Research*. 106(4):727-732.

Reidy P, Fletcher T, Shieber C, Shallcross J, Tower H, Ping M, Kenworthy L, Silman N, Aarons E. (2017). Personal protective equipment solution for UK military medical personnel working in an Ebola virus disease treatment unit in Sierra Leone. *Journal of Hospital Infection*. 96:42-48.

Rosaro M, Laverack G, Grabman LH Tripathy P, Nair N, Mwansanbo C, Azad K, Morrison J, Buhtta Z, Perry H, Rifkin S, Costello A. (2008). Community participation: lessons for maternal, newborn and child health. *Lancet*. 372(9642):962-971.

Shears P, and O'Dempsey TJ. (2015). Ebola virus disease in Africa: epidemiology and nosocomial transmission. *Journal of Hospital Infection*. 90(1):1-9.

Sridhar S. (2015). Clinical development of Ebola vaccines. *Therapeutic Advances in Vaccines*. 3 (5-6):125-138.

Sullivan NJ, Sanches A, Rollin PE, Yang Z, Nabel GJ.(2000). Development of a preventive vaccine for Ebola virus infection in primates. *Nature*. 408:606-608.

Tambo E, Chengho CF, Ugwu CE, Wurie I, Johnson J, Ngongang JY. (2017). Rebuilding transformation strategies in post-ebola epidemics in Africa. *Infectious Diseases of Poverty*. 6:71.

Tambo E, Ugwu CE, Oluwasogo AO, Isatta W, Jeannetta KJ and Jeane YN. (2015). Values and hopes of Ebola vaccines mass immunization programs and treatments adoption and implementation benefits in Africa. *International Journal of Vaccines and Vaccination*. 1(2):00011. doi:10.15406/ijvv.2015.01.00011.

Tambo, E., Ugwu, EC. and Ngogang, JY. (2014). Need of surveillance response systems to combat Ebola outbreaks in Africa countries. *Infectious Diseases of Poverty*. 3(29): doi:10.1186/2049-9957-3-29.

Tomas ME, Kundrapu S, Thota P, Sunkesula VC, Cadnum JL, Mana TS, Jencson A, O'Donnell M, Zabarsky TF, Hecker MT, Ray AT, Wilson BM, Donskey CJ.(2015). Contamination of healthcare personnel during removal of personal protective equipment. *Journal of American Medical Association Internal Medicine*. 175(12):1904-10.

United Nation Mission for Ebola Emergency Response (UNMEER)(2015). UNMEER, making a difference. The Global Ebola Response: outlook. http://ebola response.un.org.

Venkatraman N, Pedro DS, Folegatti M, Adrian V, Hill. 2018. Vaccine against Ebola virus. *Vaccine*. 36 (28):5454-5459.

Risk Communication and Community Engagement (RCCE) considerations. (2018). Ebola response in the Democratic Republic of the Congo. Geneva: World Health Organization; Licence: CCBY-NC-SA3.0IGO.

WHO (2016). Personal protective equipment for use in a filovirus disease outbreak. *Rapid advice guild line*.

Witty C, Farrar J, Ferguson N, Edmunds J, Plot P, Leach M, Davies S. (2014). Infectious disease: tough choices to reduce Ebola transmission. *Nature*. 515 (7526):192-4.

World Health Organization/SAGE MEETING (2018). Immunization, Vaccines and Biologicals. https://www.who.int/immunization/sage/ meetings/2018/april/en/.

In: Ebola Virus Disease (EVD)
Editor: Hilaire Verreau

ISBN: 978-1-53616-291-2
© 2019 Nova Science Publishers, Inc.

Chapter 3

CONTROLLING THE SPREAD OF THE EBOLA VIRUS DISEASE THROUGH THE PRISM OF HUMAN RIGHTS AND MEDICAL ETHICS

Anthony O. Nwafor[1], and Gloria C. Nwafor[2,1]*
[1]School of Law, University of Venda, South Africa
[2]Advocate of the High Court of Lesotho, South Africa

ABSTRACT

The persons infected with Ebola Virus Disease (EVD) are victims of a wide range of constraints to their human rights as protected by law. Such persons' rights are often violated because of their presumed or known EVD status, causing them to suffer both the burden of the disease and the social burden of discrimination and stigmatisation which could deter the infected persons from accessing available treatment. The victims failure or reluctance to avail themselves for treatment invariably contributes to the spreading of the disease. The work further exposes the

* Corresponding Author's E-mail: anthony.nwafor@univen.ac.za; LLB Hons (Unijos), BL, LLM (University of Nigeria), PhD (Unijos).
[1] LLB(Hons) National University of Lesotho, LLM University of Venda, South Africa, Advocate of the High Court of Lesotho.

dilemma posed by the EVD to the healthcare system, where healthcare providers are caught between the over-arching quest for self-preservation from a highly virulent disease and the professional demand of prioritising the interests of their patients over self.

1. INTRODUCTION

The world has yet again been confronted with another ominous viral infection named Ebola Virus Disease (EVD) which threatens to exterminate a significant number of human populations, especially among countries in the African region, where the potency of the disease is mostly felt. Although a significant progress has been made in containing the spread of the disease through the interventions of the international community that seek to augment the porous state of the affected African nations healthcare facilities, there are indications that addressing issues of health needs alone may not bring a closure to the incidences and the spread of EVD. Respecting the human rights of victims also holds the key in disease eradication and control as the fear of discrimination and stigmatization have the tendency to drive the victims underground and to retard the desired disclosure and sharing of information which are essential for an effective disease control and eradication.

The recognition of health as a basic human need and an enforceable right as stated in numerous national and international instruments imposes significant roles and responsibilities on the government. The global political developments following the First World War supported the move towards health as a human right. The Versailles treaty of 1919 which led to the establishment of the International Labour Organisation (ILO) emphasised the principle of "peace through social justice" and promoting social security against various hazards, including sickness and injury. The United Nations Universal Declaration of Human Rights, 1948 (Universal Declaration) states that everyone has a right to a standard of living for the health and wellbeing of himself and his family, including medical care and necessary services.[2] The constitution of the World Health Organization (WHO) which was adopted in its First World Assembly in 1946 recognises in the preamble the attainment by all peoples of the highest possible level of health and states that "Governments have responsibility for the health of their people which can be fulfilled only by the provision of adequate health and social measures".

National governments play a crucial role in the development of the health systems as part of the sovereign functions which include governance, providing health system infrastructure and training of the necessary healthcare providers.[3] Government's responsibilities in these areas of health are fulfilled through the ministries of health and other related ministries and agencies. The level of efficacy of a nation's health system is tested in times of healthcare emergencies, not merely from the efficacy of the healthcare facilities, but also from the perspective of the victims as relates to the level of accommodation and tolerance they are afforded in the prevailing healthcare emergency. Thus, in this work, the search light is focused on the human rights aspect of disease control as considered indispensable in curtailing the spread of the Ebola Virus Disease.

2. EBOLA VIRUS DISEASE (EVD): WHERE DOES IT COME FROM?

Ebola virus disease (EVD) is described, without delving into the medical intricacies of this disease, as a disease of humans and other primates caused by the Ebola virus.[4] Ebola virus is classified by virologists

---

[2] See s 25(1) of the Universal Declaration.
[3] World Health Organisation Regional Office for the Eastern Mediterranean, 'The Role of Government in Health Development Agenda item 7(a)' EM/RC53/Tech.Disc. 1, July 2006.
[4] 'Ebola virus disease' available at http://en.wikipedia.org/wiki/Ebola_virus_disease (accessed 3 September 2016); see also 'Ebola virus definition- Infectious Disease Center:Information on Infection' Medicine Net.com available at http:// www.medters.com/script/ main/ art.asp?articlekey=6518 defined Ebola virus as a notoriously deadly virus that causes fearsome symptoms, the most prominent being high fever and massive internal bleeding.

as a member of the Filoviridae viral Family of RNA viruses, which are characterized by the long, thin filaments seen in micrograph images. The virus is said to be named after the Ebola River where the virus was first discovered in the Democratic Republic of the Congo.[5]

Different types of Ebola virus have been isolated by experts in the field among which are Zaire, Sudan, and Ivory Coast Ebola virus, named after the respective countries in Africa in which the strains were found. There is also another strain of the virus called Reston Ebola virus which infects non-human primates. This was first discovered in an outbreak in Reston, Virginia, United States of America in 1989. New strains of the Ebola virus have continued to emerge. For instance, the outbreak of the disease in Bundibugyo District of Uganda in 2007 was attributed to a new strain of the virus by the US-based Center for Disease Control.[6]

The first incidence of the EVD in humans was discovered in August 1976, in Yambuku, a small rural village in Mongala District in the northern Democratic Republic of the Congo (then known as Zaire),[7] and later spread to the surrounding area in Sudan, where 284 people were infected and 151 were reported to have died.[8]

---

[5] 'Ebola Virus' available at https://microbewiki.kenyon.edu/index.php/Ebola-virus (accessed 3 September 2014); See also JH Kuhn et al. 'proposal for a revised taxonomy of the family Filoviridae: Classification, names of taxa and viruses, and virus abbreviations' (2010) 155 (12) *Archives of Virology* 2083-130.

[6] 'Ebola virus: 9 things to know about the killer disease-CNN.com August 25, 2014' available at http://edition.cnn.com/2014/08/07/world/ebola-virus-q-and-a/ (accessed 3 September 2017) where the WHO identified five different strains of the Ebola virus named after the respective areas they originated.

[7] Hewlett S Barry and Hewlett L Bonnie 'Ebola, Culture and Politics: The Anthropology of an Emerging Disease' (2007) available at http://books.google.com/books? (accessed 3 September 2017); See World Organization 'Ebola haemorrhagic fever in Zaire' 1976. Report of an International Convention. Bulletin of the World Health Organization (1978);56(2):271-29, available at http://whqlibdoc.who.int/bulletin/1978/Vol56-No2/bulletin_1978_56(2)_ 247-270.pdf (accessed 3 September 2016); see also KM Johnson, PA Webb, IV Lange, FA Murphy, 'Isolation and Characterization of a new virus(Ebola virus) causing acute haemorrhagic fever in Zaire' (1977) 1:569-71, available at http://jid.oxfordjournals.org/content/179/Supplement_1/ix.long; See also R Brown 'The virus detective who discovered Ebola in 1976'News Magazine, BBC News available at http://www.bbc.co.uk/news/magazine-28262541 (accessed 6 September 2016).

[8] 'Ebola virus disease' available at http://www.who.int/mediacentre/factsheets/fs103/en/ (accessed 5 September 2017), See World Health Organization Ebola haemorrhagic fever in Sudan (1976) Report of a World Health Organization International Study Team. Bull WHO 1978; (56):247-270 available at http://whqlibdoc.whoint/bulletin/1978/Vol56-No2/

The spread of the disease in the DRC was traced to one Mabalo Lokela, a village school headmaster, who had toured an area near the Central African Republic border along the Ebola River between 12-22 August 1976. He died of Ebola disease on the 8 of September, 1976 barely three weeks after the manifestations of the symptoms of the disease. A number of other cases were subsequently reported, and almost all were centered on the Yambuku mission hospital where the index case had received medical attention, and others who had contacts with infected persons. A total of 318 cases of infection resulting in 280 deaths, 88% fatality rate, were recorded at the time in the DRC.[9]

The initial outbreak of the disease in the DRC was contained with the help of the World Health Organization in collaboration with the Congolese air force who ensured the quarantining of infected villagers and isolated suspected cases, sterilizing medical equipment, and providing protective clothing.[10] The virus responsible for the outbreak of the disease in the DRC was initially thought to be the Marburg virus[11] but was later identified as a new type of virus related to Marburg, and named after the nearby Ebola River.[12]

As a contact disease, the spread could be quite rapid and unassuming as witnessed in those African nations where the incidences of the disease were recorded. The healthcare providers who came in contact with bodily fluids from the infected persons were also infected. Incidents such as these founded justification for some healthcare providers like doctors and nurses showing reluctance and lack of professionalism in dealing with people

---

bulletin_1978_56(2)_247_270.pdf (accessed 5 September 2014). See also RT Emond, B Evans, ET Bowen, et al 'A case of Ebola virus infection' (1977) 2 British Medical Journal 541-544.

[9] JW King, 'Ebola Virus' (2008) eMedicine, WebMd available at http://www.emedicine.com/ MED/topic626.htm (assessed 5 September 2014).

[10] See *'Ebola Virus Disease'* available at http://en.wikipedia.org/wiki/Ebola_virus_disease (accessed 3 September 2014).

[11] Marburg virus is a haemorrhagic fever virus of the Filoviridae family of viruses, first noticed and described during small epidemics in the German cities Marburg and Frankfurt and the Yugoslav capital Belgrade in the 1960s; See JH Kuhn et al 'proposal for a revised taxonomy of the family Filoviridae: Classification, names of taxa and viruses, and virus abbreviations' (2010) 155 (12) *Archives of Virology* 103.

[12] 'Ebola virus disease' available at http://www.who.int/mediacentre/factsheets/fs103/en/ (accessed 5 September 2014).

infected with EVD.[13] But such conducts by those healthcare service providers can only aggravate rather than eradicate the spread of the disease. The signs are already being felt in the DRC where the resurgence of the disease has been reported with about 500 infected persons and no less than half of that number are said to have died in spite of the newly discovered vaccine which has shown some potency in the treatment of the infected persons.[14] The spread of the disease is yet to be contained as a recent report suggests that the number of the infected persons in the DRC has now reached 2000 is continuing to escalate.[15] Uganda, which shares border with the DRC is now on record as having encoundered the spread of the virus. A 5-year-old Congolese boy was diagnosed with the virus in Uganda. The government in that country is shown to be proactive in containing the spread of the disease having trained a sizeable number of health workers and provided health facilities for easy diagnosis and treatment of the infected persons, arrangements which are reported to have so far assisted in curtailing the spread of the disease in that country.[16] Those logistics have not, however, prevented the death of the 5-year-old child whose grandmother and younger brother have also been infected by the disease.[17]

---

[13] 'Ebola Patients Abandoned, Health Team Down Tools- Health' *Nairaland* available at http://www.nairaland.com/1862229/ebola-patients-abondoned-health-team (accessed 9 September 2014).

[14] Jon Cohen, 'Ebola Vaccine is having a 'major impact' but worries about Congo outbreak grow" available at https://www.sciencemag.org/news/2018/12/ebola-vaccine-having-major-impact-outbreak-may-still-explode-west-africa (accessed on 12 December 2018).

[15] A more recent report indicated that there are more than 2,100 cases and 1,412 confirmed deaths, and that the outbreak in the eastern DRC is the second largest in history. It has a 67% fatality rate and 11 months after it began, the case numbers are still escalating. It is disproportionately affecting women (55% of cases) and children (28%). The WHO says the national and regional risk levels are very high and containment of the spread to North Kivu and Ituri provinces is unlikely, unless a break in the fighting makes it safe for health workers. See Sarah Boseley and Jason Burke, 'Terrifying' Ebola epidemic out of control in DRC, say experts' available at https://www.theguardian.com/world/2019/may/15/ebola-in-the-drc-everything-you-need-to-know (accessed on 10 July 2019).

[16] Richard Greene and Debra Goldschmidt, 'Ebola outbreak spreads outside Congo, WHO says' available at https://edition.cnn.com/2019/06/11/health/ebola-outside-congo-uganda-africa-bn/index.html (accessed on 10 July 2019).

[17] DR Congo Ebola Outbreak: Child in Uganda dies of virus' available at https://www.bbc.com/news/world-africa-48603273 (accessed 10 July 2019).

The recent outbreak of the disease in the DRC is reported as the 10th of such experience since 1976.[18] Multiplicity of factors are shown to militate against effective control of the disease in the DRC. Many Ebola deaths are never reported. Decades of conflict have led to widespread mistrust of the authorities. Some deny the disease exists, believing it to be a poison invented by the international community to traffic body parts. Others do not trust trained medical staff to look after the sick. There are those who simply do not want their loved ones snatched from them, sealed up in a plastic body bag and buried anonymously by someone else.[19] In the prevailing situation, said Laurence Sailly, MSF emergency coordinator in Beni, "people might have no other choice than to seek medical help in health facilities that do not have adequate triage or infection prevention and control measures in place, which makes the risk of contamination higher."[20]

It would seem that medical approach which vaccination is associated with, (the stockpile of which is reported to be presently inadequate to contain the spread of the disease in the DRC alone),[21] may not sole handedly attain the desired result of eradicating the spread of the virus. A complemental legal approach which is galvanized by the precepts of human rights protection is inevitable. The victims must have all required assurances of protection of their confidentiality, protection against discrimination and stigmatization among others, that are usually attendant

---

[18] Ibid.

[19] James Landale, 'Ebola in DR Congo: Fear and mistrust stalk battle to halt outbreak' available at https://www.bbc.com/news/world-africa-48908993 (accessed on 10 July 2019).

[20] Medecins Sans Frontieres, 'Ebola Outbreak in DRC: Fighting an epidemic in a conflict zone' available at https://www.doctorswithoutborders.org/ebola-outbreak-drc (accessed 10 July 2019).

[21] Stephanie Soucheray 'As Ebola rages on, DRC sees more displaced people' available at http://www.cidrap.umn.edu/news-perspective/2019/07/ebola-rages-drc-sees-more-displaced-people (accessed 10 July 2019), reported that one of the scientists who helped develop Merck's rVSV-ZEBOV vaccine said there was not currently enough vaccine stockpiled to successfully stop this outbreak.In an interview with the Canadian Broadcast Company (CDC), microbiologist Gary Kobinger, PhD, said the stockpile of the vaccine needs to reach 1 million doses, and halting the virus would require about 72% of the population to be immunized.

the disclosure of such pandemic especially in the developing nations, to enable them accede to any available medical solution.

3. MEDICAL ETHICS AND THE LAW

The practice of medicine as a profession is highly regulated. Men and women involved in that practice do on daily basis come across patients' information which are strictly confidential. The quest to curtail abuses of such confidence and to ensure optimal exercise of dexterity by the physician in the care for his or her patient necessitated the formulation of some moral code of conduct, some of which have over the years metamorphosed into rules of law, to serve as guides in directing the services of the physician to his or her patient.[22] These bodies of moral rules are simply referred to as the ethics of the profession or rules of professional conduct. The earliest of such medical ethics is embodied in a statement attributed to a great physician, Hippocrates, who at present times is referred to as the father of modern medicine, and whose statement is administered as an Oath to practitioners of medicine at the point of their admission into the profession.[23] The Hippocratic Oath states in part as follows:

> I swear …that, according to my ability and judgment, I will keep this Oath and this contract:...Into whatever homes I go, I will enter them for the benefit of the sick, avoiding any voluntary act of impropriety or corruption,....Whatever I see or hear in the lives of my patients, whether in connection with my professional practice or not, which ought not to be spoken of outside, I will keep secret, as considering all such things to be private. So long as I maintain this Oath faithfully and without corruption, may it be granted to me to partake of life fully and the practice of my art, gaining the respect of all men for all time. However, should I transgress this Oath and violate it, may the opposite be my fate.[24]

---

[22] A. O. Nwafor 'Comparative perspectives on euthanasia in Nigeria and Ethiopia' (2010) 18 (2) *African Journal of International and Comparative Law* 178.

[23] Ibid.

[24] 'The Hippocratic Oath' available at http://www.nlm.nih.gov/hmd/greek/greek_oath.html (accessed 18 April 2015).

The World Medical Association has made some modifications to this Oath to bring it in line with the practice and language of modern medicine but without losing the precepts. The modified version, otherwise referred to as the Geneva Declaration of 1949, enjoins the physician to maintain utmost respect for human life from time of conception, even under threat, and not to use his medical knowledge contrary to the laws of humanity.[25]

Healthcare providers operate on a foundation of ethical principles, namely beneficence (doing good), non-maleficence (do no harm), and justice (just distribution of finite resources).[26] Beneficence is the most prominent principle that comes into play in considering the treatment of patients infected by the Ebola virus. Beneficence demands from the healthcare provider some elements of empathy in relating with the patient, so long as the patient's initial complaint falls within the provider's scope of practice.[27] The failure by the healthcare provider to observe that precept is inconsistent with the ethical principles of beneficence. The risk of disease transmission, the grounds on which healthcare providers are most likely to refuse to treat the Ebola patients, does not preclude healthcare providers from upholding the principles enshrined in the concept of beneficence. Under this ethical medical principle, healthcare providers are under obligation to attend to patients with infectious disease.[28] The basis of ethics, according to Swami Vivekananda, is to become more and more selfless: "Whether men understand it or not, they are impelled by that power behind to become unselfish. That is the foundation of morality. It is the quintessence of all ethics, preached in any language, or any religion, or

---

[25] Nwafor, op cit p. 179.

[26] 'Are Healthcare Providers Legally Obligated to Treat Ebola Patients?' available at http://midlevelu.com/blog/are-healthcare-providers-legally-obligated-treat-ebola-patients (accessed 19 April 2015).

[27] Ibid.

[28] Are Healthcare Providers Legally Obligated to Treat Ebola Patients? available at http://www.midlevelu.com/blog/are-healcare-providers-legally-obligated-treat-ebola-patients (accessed 4 February 2015); see also The Hippocratic Oath www.med.uottawa.ca/students/md/.../eng/hippocratic_oath.html The primary standard of care for all healthcare professionals is the delivery of high quality care to everyone, regardless of underlying disease, failure to do so is a potential breech of medical ethics available at http://health.ri.gov/publications/briefs/ 20141007ProfessionalResponsibilities ForTreatmentOfPatientsWithEbola.pdf (accessed 7 February 2015).

by any prophet in the world. Be thou unselfish", Not 'I', but 'Thou - that is the background of ethical codes."[29]

In the African nations that have witnessed the spread of Ebola, healthcare providers were reported to have abandoned the victims in preference for the preservation of self. Respite only came to the victims with the intervention of mostly international volunteer organisations some of whose personnel actually paid with their lives to save the Ebola victims.[30] Although this may seem infinitesimal when considered along with the hordes of other reasons that galvanized the spread of the disease such as, the lateness and narrow scope of the public-health campaigns at the inception of the disease, literacy rate in the countries that were mostly affected, the spreading of false rumor about the disease, economic poverty and porous healthcare system in the affected countries, lack of disease surveillance networks in the affected countries, slow response by the international community and the interconnectivity and free movement of persons along international boundaries,[31] mistrust of officials, foreigners and security challenges in the DRC at least,[32] the focus on self-preservation negates the underlying ethical obligation of the physician which demands the denial of self in preference for the patient's interest. The recommended practice in the medical profession is that a practitioner who is exposed to health risk should adopt the necessary measures to protect self, apart from abandoning patient. In the context of Ebola or any other infectious disease, the health care provided is expected to wear protective clothing, including masks, gloves, gowns, and eye protection.[33]

---

[29] C S Shah, 'Revival of medical Ethics' available www.boloji.com/ index.cfm?md= Content&sd=Articles&ArticleID (accessed 4 February 2015).

[30] 'Should doctors "have" to treat Ebola patients? - AMERICAblog available at americablog.com/2014/09/doctors-treat-ebola-patients.html (accessed 24 March 2016).

[31] Julia Belluz, "Seven reasons why this Ebola epidemic spun out of control" available at https://www.vox.com/2014/9/4/6103039/Seven-reasons-why-this-ebola-virus-outbreak-epidemic-out-of-control (accessed 15/12/2018).

[32] See 'Ebola in the DRC: everything you need to know' available at https://www.theguardian.com/world/2019/may/15/ebola-in-the-drc-everything-you-need-to-know (accessed 09/07/2019).

[33] Centers for Disease Control and Prevention, 'Ebola in Democratic Republic of Congo' available at https://wwwnc.cdc.gov/travel/notices/alert/ebola-democratic-republic-of-the-congo (accessed 10 July 2019).

4. PATIENT CARE AND HUMAN RIGHTS

Patient care refers to the prevention, treatment, and management of illness and the preservation of physical and mental well-being through services offered by health professionals.[34] More specifically, patient care consists of services rendered by health professionals (or non-professionals under their supervision) for the benefit of patients.[35] Patient care is a discrete and important aspect of the right to healthcare that merits attention and scrutiny as a human right issue.[36]

Human rights in patient care refers, not just to entitlements for actual patients, but to legal, ethical, and human rights standards in the provision of care that concern health providers and the entire community.[37] Apart from the ethical standard which demands that healthcare providers should place the interests of the patient above personal interests, it is internationally recognised that patients are by law entitled to some basic empowerment rights such as information, consent, free choice, privacy and confidentiality, rights to a remedy for abuses, and rights of access to services, in the course of their dealings with the healthcare providers.[38] These components of human rights constitute a critical part of the provision of quality and appropriate healthcare aimed at attaining the highest standard of health.

The call for the protection of patients' rights is a movement that is growing globally to make governments and healthcare providers more accountable for providing access to quality healthcare services.[39] Patients'

---

[34] Patient care - definition of Patient care by Medical dictionary available at medical-dictionary.thefreedictionary.com/Patient+care (accessed 21 January 2015).

[35] 'Health and Human Rights Resource Guide' Harvard School of Public Heath: Harvard University available at http://hhrguide.org/wp-content/uploads/sites/25/2014/03/ HHRRG-master.pdf (accessed 12 January 2015).

[36] Jonathan Cohen and Tamar Ezer 'Human Rights in Patients Care: A Theoretical and Practical Framework' (2015) 15(2) *Health and Human Rights* 7.

[37] 'Health and Human Rights' A Resource Guide for the Open Society Institute and Soros Foundations Network June 2007 available *at* http://kelinkenya.org/wp-content/uploads/2010/10/Health-and-Human-Rights-Resource-Guide-OSI-Equitas.pdf (accessed 25 January 2015).

[38] Ibid.

[39] 'Health and Human Rights' A Resource Guide for the Open Society Institute and Soros Foundations Network June 2007 available at http://kelinkenya.org/wp-content/uploads/

rights are an integral component of human rights. They promote and sustain beneficial relationships between patients and healthcare providers. The role of the patients' rights therefore is to reaffirm fundamental human rights in the healthcare context by according patients humane treatment. The need to protect and promote the dignity, integrity, and respect of all patients is now widely accepted.[40] To this end, the WHO predicts that the articulation of patients' rights will in turn make people more conscious of their responsibilities when seeking and receiving or providing healthcare. This will ensure that patient-provider relationships are marked by mutual support and respect.[41]

Patients' rights vary in different countries and in different jurisdictions, often depending upon the prevailing cultural and social norms. Different models of the patient-physician relationship—which can also represent the citizen-state relationship—have evolved. These have informed the particular rights to which patients are entitled. In North America and Europe, for instance, there are at least four models which depict this relationship, namely: the paternalistic model, the informative model, the interpretive model, and the deliberative model. Each of these suggests different professional obligations of the physician toward the patient. For instance, in the paternalistic model, the best interests of the patient as judged by the clinical expert are valued above the provision of comprehensive medical information and decision-making power to the patient. The informative model, by contrast, sees the patient as a consumer who is in the best position to judge what is in her own interest, and thus views the doctor as chiefly a provider of information. There continues to be enormous debate about how best to conceive of this relationship, but there is also growing international consensus that all patients, including those infected with Ebola, have a fundamental right to privacy, to the

2010/10/Health-and-Human-Rights-Resource-Guide-OSI-Equitas.pdf (accessed 25 January 2015).

[40] Benson Oduor Ojwang, Emily Atieno Oguta and Peter Maina Matu 'Nurses' impoliteness as an impediment to patients' rights in selected Kenyan hospital' (2010) 12 (2) *Health and Human Rights* 101.

[41] Karima Ahmed Elsayed, Omebrahiem A El-Melegy and Amaal M El-Zeftawy 'The Effect of an Educational Intervention on Nurses' Awareness about Patients' Rights in Tanta' (2013) 9(9) *Journal of American Science* 211.

confidentiality of their medical information, to consent or to refuse treatment, and to be informed about relevant risk to them of medical procedures.[42]

A vast and severe range of human rights violations occur in the process of patients care. In response to the growing concerns about these abuses of patients' rights in many parts of the world, the concept of 'human rights in patient care' evolved as a framework for monitoring healthcare providers, analysing abuses and holding accountable the violators of such rights.[43] Respect for patient's dignity and autonomy are the keys to a cordial relationship between the healthcare provider and the patient.

5. HUMAN RIGHTS OF PEOPLE INFECTED WITH EVD

The term human rights may be used either in the abstract or philosophical sense, to denote a special kind of moral claim that all humans may invoke, or more pragmatically, as the manifestation of these claims in positive law, for example as constitutional guarantees that serve as the basis to hold governments accountable under national legal processes.[44]

Human rights are in some circles discussed, albeit erroneously, as synonymous with constitutional rights. This perhaps stems from the general perception that every right is enforceable in law. The word 'right' means that to which a person has a just and valid claim, whether it be land, a thing, or the privilege of doing or saying something. 'Human' pertains to having characteristics of, or the nature of mankind. Human rights are thus rights which all persons (mankind), everywhere, and at all times, have by

---

[42] 'WHO| Patients rights' available at http://www.who.int/genomics/public/patientrights/en/ (accessed 23 January 2015).

[43] Cohen op cit p. 7.

[44] Frans Viljoen, *International Human Rights Law in Africa 2nd ed* (United Kingdom: Oxford University Press, 2012) p 3. See also David P Forsythe, *Human Rights in International Relations* 2nd ed (New York: Cambridge University Press, 2006) p. 3 where human rights are widely considered to be those fundamental moral rights of the person that are necessary for a life with dignity and as the means to a greater social end; the legal system that tells us at any given point in time which rights are considered most fundamental in society.

virtue of being mortal and rational creatures. They are inherent in every human being by virtue of their humanity.[45] They are fundamental rights owned by every human being and are defined in national and international human rights instruments and codes.[46] When human rights have been ratified and acceded to in international agreements or legislated for in national legal systems, they also become legal rights.[47]

The Universal Declaration of Human Rights which was proclaimed by the United Nations General Assembly in December 1948 is historically the foundational instrument upon which various human rights legislation are predicated. The influence of the Universal Declaration on later international and national instruments and law has been so far- reaching that it has been variously described as the "Magna Carta of the world, the cornerstone of United Nations and a common language for all humanity."[48] The Universal Declaration has as one of its objectives, the recognition of the inherent dignity, equal and inalienable rights of all members of the human family as the foundation of freedom, justice and peace in the world.[49]

The provision of adequate healthcare for the citizens by the state is a fundamental human right which is indispensable to the realization and exercise of other human rights. Every human being is entitled to the enjoyment of the highest attainable standard of health conducive to living a life in dignity. Article 25(1) of the Universal Declaration provides that "everyone has the right to a standard of living adequate for the health and well-being of himself and of his family, including food, clothing, housing and medical care and necessary social services".[50] Although the Universal

---

[45] A.O. Nwafor 'Enforcing Fundamental Rights in Nigerian Courts-Processes and Challenges' (2009) 4 *African Journal of Legal Studies* 1.

[46] Ames Dhai and David McQuoid- Mason, *Bioethics, Human Rights and Health: Law, Principle and Practice* (Cape Town: Juta & Co Ltd, 2011) p. 36.

[47] Ibid.

[48] S Iwuagwu (ed) *HIV/AIDS and Human Rights: Role of the Judiciary* (Nigeria: CRH Publication 2001) p. 50.

[49] See the Preamble to the Universal Declaration of Human Rights 1984 (Universal Declaration).

[50] Universal Declaration of Human Rights, General Assembly Resolution 217A(111)10th December 1948.

Declaration is not a treaty, it has been widely accepted.[51] The norms therein declared have metamorphosed into customary international law. Indeed, almost all the norms contained in the Universal Declaration have been transmuted into binding standards in the International Convention on Civil and Political Rights (ICCPR) and International Convention on Economic, Social and Cultural Rights (ICESCR).

The right to healthcare of people infected with EVD is particularly susceptible to violations in the healthcare settings especially where there are inadequate healthcare facilities to address situations of health emergencies. For instance, it was reported that in Nigeria the healthcare providers abandoned Ebola patients and walked away from an Ebola treatment Center (the Infectious Disease Hospital) in Yaba, Lagos. The healthcare providers allegedly claimed that they abandoned the patients because of what they perceived as the lack-lustre attitude of their country's health officials to the plight of the Ebola patients who were quarantined at the Center. The Ebola patients were reportedly housed in a dilapidated and abandoned building at the Center without quality care, functioning water supply and no air conditioning facilities. The families of the patients took the responsibilities for the medical needs of the patients.[52] The failure or neglect to provide for the needs of the patient in such circumstances amounts to an infringement by the healthcare providers of the right to healthcare of the patient.

In Liberia, Guinea, and Sierra Leone the victims of the disease were quarantined in make-shift shelters without adequate provisions of treatment facilities and other amenities of life.[53] Restrictions were also imposed on individual's houses, neighbourhoods, villages, and in some cases the entire

---

[51] Ebenezer Durojaye and Olabisi Ayankogbe, 'A rights- based approach to access to HIV treatment in Nigeria' (2005) 5 *African Human Rights Law Journal* 289.

[52] Ebola Patients Abandoned, Health Team Down Tools- Health- Nairaland' available at http://www.nairaland.com/1862229/ebola-patients-abondoned-health-team (accessed 9 September 2014); See also 'Nigeria Hasn't Given Priority To Ebola Treatment, Abandons Nano Silver Treatment' available at http://www.nursingworldnigeria.com/2014/08/nigeria-hasn-rsquo-t-given-priority-to-e (accessed 9 September 2016).

[53] 'Ebola virus disease' available at http://en.wikipedia.org/wiki/Ebola_virus_disease (accessed 9 September 2017).

administrative districts.[54] All these were done under the guise of preventing the spread of the disease in those communities. The quarantining of persons in healthcare related emergencies is expected to comply with certain criteria as prescribed under the international human rights law which indicates that "restrictions on human rights in the name of public health or public emergency meet requirements of legality, evidence-based necessity, and proportionality. Restrictions such as quarantine or isolation of symptomatic individuals must, at a minimum, be provided for and carried out in accordance with the law. They must be strictly necessary to achieve a legitimate objective, be the least intrusive and restrictive available means to reach the objective, based on scientific evidence, neither arbitrary nor discriminatory in application, of limited duration, respectful of human dignity, and subject to review. When quarantines are imposed, governments have absolute obligation to ensure access to food, water, and healthcare."[55] The observance of these internationally laid down procedure provides some assurance to the affected persons that the restrictions temporarily imposed on their freedoms are for their own good and for the protection of the public interests and not punishment for being victims or potential victims of the infectious disease.

The need for respect for the human rights of victims of the EVD would be better appreciated when articulated from the perspective of the doctor and patient relationship. From ancient times, physicians have recognized that the health and wellbeing of patients depend upon a collaborative effort between physician and the patient. Patients share with doctors the responsibility for their own healthcare. The patient-physician relationship is of greatest benefit to the patients when they bring medical problems to the attention of their physicians in a timely fashion, provide information about their medical condition to the best of their ability, and work with their physician in a mutual alliance.[56] The physician-patient relationship is

---

[54] 'West Africa: Respect Rights in Ebola Response| Human Rights Watch' available at http://www.hrw.org/news/2014/09/15/west-africa-respect-rights-ebola-response (accessed 22 September 2017).

[55] Ibid.

[56] 'Opinion 10.01-Fundamental Elements of the patient-Physician Relationship' available at www.ama-assn.org/ama/pub/physician.../medical.../opinion1001.page (accessed 4 February

central to the practice of healthcare and is essential for the delivery of high-quality healthcare in the diagnosis and treatment of disease.[57] The relationship of a physician and a patient is based on trust and gives rise to physician' ethical obligations to place patient's welfare above his/her own self-interest and above obligations to other groups, and to advocate for the patient's welfare. It is the type of relationship described as fiduciary.[58]

Although the term fiduciary may not have enjoyed specific definition, its precepts are not so difficult to grasp. In *Bristol and West Building Society v Mothew*[59] Millett LJ was convinced that a fiduciary is "someone who has undertaken to act for or on behalf of another in a particular matter in circumstances which give rise to a relationship of trust and confidence." The central idea is that a fiduciary is an actor who is "required to look after the interest(s) of....others with vigilance, dedication and selflessness."[60] A fiduciary duty entails abnegation of self interest in preference for loyalty and the protection of others. The limits of the expectations on a fiduciary are discernible in *Mothew's case* where Millett LJ stated that:

> The various obligations of a fiduciary merely reflect different aspects of his core duties of loyalty and fiduciary. Breach of fiduciary obligation, therefore, connotes disloyalty or infidelity. Mere incompetence is not

---

2015); The patients' satisfaction with an encounter with healthcare services is mainly dependent on the duration and efficiency of care, and how empathetic and communicative the healthcare providers are. It is favoured by a good physician –patient relationship. Also, patients who are well informed of the necessary procedures in a clinical encounter, and the time it is expected to take, are generally more satisfied even if there is a longer waiting time see Michael Pulia 'Simple Tips to Improve Patients Satisfaction' (2011) 18 (1) American Academy of Emergency Medicine 18-19.

[57] 'Doctor-patient relationship' available at http://en.wikipedia.org/wiki/ Doctor%E2% 80% 93patient_relationship (accessed 14 January 2015).

[58] SB Odunsi and AO Nwafor 'Medical Confidentiality: Right of HIV/AIDS Patient and the Third Party Interest' (2006) 16 (2) *Lesotho Law Journal* 250.

[59] [1998] Ch 1 at 18A.

[60] Moe Litman, 'Fiduciary law in the hospital context: the prescriptive duty of protective intervention' (2007) 15 Health Law Journal 299. See also *Bristol and West Building Society v Mothew* [1998] Ch 1 at 18A; *Ultraframe (UK) Ltd v Fielding* [2005] EWHC 1638 (Ch) para 1300. In *Extrasure Travel Insurance Ltd v Scattergood* [2003] 1 BCLC 598 at 617 Mr Jonathan Crow stated that fiduciary duties are concerned with concepts of honesty and loyalty and not with competence.

enough. A servant who loyally does his incompetent best for his master is not unfaithful and is not guilty of a breach of fiduciary duty.[61]

In the medical context, a physician that has lived up to the standard of an average practitioner in the field would not be condemned merely because the desired result was not attained. In order for the physician to make accurate diagnosis and provide optimal treatment recommendation, the patient should communicate all relevant information about an illness or injury. This may require the disclosure of sensitive information, which would be embarrassing or harmful in some cases, if they were known to third parties. The promise of confidentiality permits the patient to trust that information revealed to the physician will not be further disseminated. The expectation of confidentiality derives from the public oath which the physician has taken, and from the accepted code of professional ethics.[62] Physicians are generally obliged to refrain from divulging information which their patients have passed to them in confidence to third parties.[63]

5.1. Ebola Victims and Right to Dignity

Human dignity refers to one's self-esteem, self-regard and self-respect. Dignity is concerned with how individuals feel, think and behave in relation to the worth or value of themselves and others. To treat persons with dignity is to treat them as being of worth, in a way that is respectful of their diversity, as valued individuals.[64] When a person's dignity is interfered with, the person feels degraded, embarrassed and humiliated.[65] On the contrary, when dignity is respected, persons feel in control, valued,

---

[61] *Mothew's case* p. 18E-F.

[62] JO Mary Ludwig and Wylie Burke 'Physician –Patient Relationship' University of Washington School of Medicine, Ethics in Medicine available at http://depts..washington.edu/bioethx/topics/physpt.html (accessed 14 January 2017).

[63] Odunsi & Nwafor op cit p. 250.

[64] Dignity and me – RCN, available at www.rcn.org.uk › ... › CPD online learning › Dignity in health care (accessed 19 July 2017).

[65] Annabel Burt 'What is the relationship between human rights and human dignity' available at www.peterjepson.com/law/CIT2-6%20Burt.pdf (accessed 14 April 2015).

confident, comfortable and able to make decisions for themselves.[66] In healthcare situations, dignity may be promoted or diminished by the physical environment; organisational culture; by the attitudes and behaviour of healthcare providers and others and by the way in which care activities are carried out. Healthcare providers are under obligation to treat all patients in all settings and of any health status with dignity, and dignified care should continue after death.[67]

The Universal Declaration of Human Rights was pivotal in popularizing the use of 'dignity' or 'human dignity' in human rights discourse.[68] The importance of respect for human dignity as a human right draws from the events proceeding and up to the Second World War where millions of Jews were used for human experiment, tortured and killed by agents of Adolf Hitler. The world was alarmed by the horrendous dehumanisation of humanity in the torture chambers created by Hitler. This galvanised global action leading to the recognition of the need for the protection of human dignity by the United Nations.[69]

The UN Universal Declaration of Human Rights which embodies a universally accepted framework for the protection of human rights recognizes that the inherent dignity and the equal and inalienable rights of all members of the human family are the foundations of freedom, justice and peace in the world. Article 1 of the Universal Declaration states that all human beings are born free and equal in dignity and in rights.[70] The Universal Declaration links dignity with other fundamental rights. Article 22 provides that everyone, as a member of society, has the right to social security and is entitled to realization, through national effort and international co-operation and in accordance with the organization and

---

[66] Dignity and me – RCN www.rcn.org.uk › ... › *CPD online learning* › *Dignity in health care* (accessed 19 July 2017).

[67] Ibid

[68] Christopher McCrudden 'Human Dignity and Judicial Interpretation of Human Rights' (2008) 19 Issue 4 European Journal of International Law 655-724.

[69] Annabel Burt 'What is the relationship between human rights and human dignity' available at www.peterjepson.com/law/CIT2-6%20Burt.pdf (accessed 12 June 2018).

[70] Universal Declaration of Human Rights, General Assembly Resolution 217A(111) 10th December 1948.

resources of each State, of the economic, social and cultural rights indispensable for his dignity and the free development of his personality.

Various other international and national human rights instruments have followed the lead by the Universal Declaration in upholding the inextricable relationship between human rights and human dignity. The ICESCR states in its preamble that human rights derive from the inherent dignity of the human person. The ICCPR recognizes that all human rights derive from the inherent dignity of the human person. Article 10 of the ICCPR provides that all persons deprived of liberty shall be treated with humanity and with respect for the inherent dignity of the human person. The African Charter contains provisions recognizing the right to dignity in article 5 which states that every individual shall have the right to the respect of the dignity inherent in a human being and to the recognition of his legal status. All forms of exploitation and degradation of man, particularly slavery, slave trade, torture, cruel, inhuman or degrading punishment and treatment shall be prohibited.

The respective national constitutions of countries affected by the outbreak of the EVD including Nigeria, Serra Leone, Democratic Republic of the Congo, Liberian and Guinea, recognize the inherent dignity of the human person. Section 34(1) of the Nigerian Constitution specifically provides that every individual is entitled to respect for the dignity of his person, and as such prohibits the subjecting of individuals to torture or to inhuman or degrading treatment; slavery or servitude; and to perform forced or compulsory labour.[71] The constitution of the Republic of Guinea is even more forceful in its pronouncement on the dignity of human person. Article 5 of the Constitution declares that "[t]he human person and their dignity are sacred. The State has the duty to respect them and to protect them."[72] Similarly, the Constitution of the DRC declares in Article 11 that all human beings are born free and equal in dignity and rights. Article 16 provides that the individual is sacred. The State has the obligation to respect and protect him/her. All persons have the right to life,

---

[71] Similar provisions are contained in ss 19 and 20 of the Sierra Leonean Constitution of 1991, and article 12 of the Liberian Constitution.

[72] See also article 6 of the Constitution which prohibits torture, inhuman and degrading treatment.

physical integrity and to the free development of their personality, while respecting the law, public order, the rights of others and public morality. No one may be held in slavery or in a similar condition. No one may be subject to cruel, inhumane or degrading treatment. No one may be submitted to forced or compulsory labor.[73]

Although the constitutions of Sierra Leone and Liberia respectively did not expressly use the word 'dignity' in their provisions, the prohibitions of torture, inhuman and degrading treatment as provided in those constitutions are obviously aimed at the protection of human dignity. Inferences could be drawn from the South African courts pronouncements to buttress this point. In *S v Makwanyane*[74] O' Regan J stated that "[r]ecognising a right to dignity is an acknowledgement of the intrinsic worth of human beings: human beings are entitled to be treated as worthy of respect and concern. This right therefore is the foundation of many of other rights that are specifically entrenched [in the Bill of Rights]". In *Le Roux and Others v Dey*[75] Harms DP observed that:

> The term 'dignity' covers a number of concepts in... the Constitution, but in the present context we are concerned with the plaintiff's sense of self-worth. Melius de Villiers spoke of inborn right to the tranquil enjoyment of one's peace of mind and the valued serene condition in one's social or individual life which has been violated when one is subjected to offensive and degrading treatment, or exposed to ill-will, radicle, disesteem or contempt.

In the consolidated cases of *Dawood and Another v Minister of Home Affairs and Others, Shalabi and Another v Minister of Home Affairs and Others, Thomas and Another v Minister of Home Affairs and Others*[76] Corbett CJ stated that under the South Africa constitutional order, the recognition and protection of human dignity is the foundational

---

[73] See The Constitution of the Democratic Republic of the Congo, 2005, adopted by the National Assembly on May 13, 2005, and approved by the Congolese people by the referendum of December 18 and 19, 2005.
[74] 1995 (3) SA 391 (CC) para 328.
[75] 2010 (4) SA 210 (SCA) para 20.
[76] 2000 (3) SA 936 (CC) para 35.

constitutional value. Descending to the inhuman treatment of the black population during the apartheid era, the judge observed that:

> The value of dignity in our constitutional framework cannot... be doubted. The Constitution asserts dignity to contradict our past in which human dignity for black South Africans was routinely and cruelly denied. It asserts it too to inform the future, to invest in our democracy respect for the intrinsic worth of all human beings. Human dignity therefore informs constitutional adjudication and interpretation at a range of levels.

Dignity has thus been described as the *grundnorm* of the South African Constitution.[77] Patients have equal worth as every other human being irrespective of the nature of the disease which the person is afflicted. Victims should be treated as persons able to feel, think and behave in relation to their own worth or value. Although Ebola is classified as an epidemic, the victims should not be treated as outcasts in the society. Conveying a victim of Ebola in a wheel barrow or being dumped in a house or abandoned at make-shift healthcare centre as reported in some countries at the initial outbreak of the EVD are all acts of infringement on the victims' right to dignity.[78] Even the dead should be buried with dignity and not cast into the 'evil forest' as accursed persons only fit as food for animals, practices which were recorded in some countries at the inception of the epidemic.[79]

---

[77] See Druccila Cornell, Stu Woolman, Sam Fuller, Jason Brickhill, Michael Bishop and Diana Dunbar, *The Dignity Jurisprudence of the Constitutional Court of South Africa* Vol I (New York, Fordam University Press, 2013) 7.

[78] Man transports a possible victim of the Ebola virus in a wheelbarrow on Thursday at the Ebola treatment center at Island Hospital in Monrovia, Liberia. (Oct 2, 2014.) *Available at* http://earthsquare.net/7759 (accessed 15 May 2015); See also 'Ebola Patients Abandoned, Health Team Down Tools- Health' *Nairaland* available at http://www.nairaland.com/1862229/ebola-patients-abondoned-health-team (accessed 9 September 2014).

[79] Matthew Blake, "Dogs eating corpses of Ebola victims in Liberia" Mail Online available at https://www.dailymail.co.uk/news/article-2737684/Dogs-EATING-corpses-Ebola-victims-Liberia-health-teams-pile-bodies-shallow-grave-middle-night-locals-refused-permission-use-land.html (accessed 15 December, 2018).

5.2. Ebola Victims and the Right to Information

The right to information is an internationally recognised human right. It applies to every person who seeks to receive or impart information on a subject matter of interest. The ICCPR recognizes the right to information in article 19(2) which provides that everyone shall have the right to freedom of expression; this right shall include freedom to seek, receive and impart information and ideas of all kinds, regardless of frontiers, either orally, in writing or in print, in the form of art, or through any other media of his choice. In relation to women, article 10(h) of CEDAW enjoins state parties to provide access to specific educational information to ensure the health and well-being of families, including information and advice on family planning. Article 9(1) of the African Charter provides that every individual shall have the right to receive information. More specific provisions on health related information are found in the Convention on Human Rights and Biomedicine which provides in article 10(2) that everyone is entitled to know any information collected about his or her health.[80] The World Medical Association's Declaration of Lisbon on Rights of the Patient (Lisbon Declaration) states that the patient has the right to receive information about himself/herself recorded in any of his/her medical records, and to be fully informed about his/her health status including the medical facts about his/her condition.[81] A patient's right to be informed constitutes an essential part of healthcare accessibility.[82]

In many cases, patients, except perhaps the few enlightened ones, are often unaware of their rights, including the right to information on their

---

[80] Convention for the Protection of Human Rights and Dignity of the Human Being with regard to the Application of Biology and Medicine: Convention on Human Rights and Biomedicine Oviedo, 4.IV. 1997 available at http://conventions.coe.int/Treaty/en/Treaties/Html/164.htm (accessed 25 June 2018).

[81] The Declaration of Lisbon was adopted in 1981 by the 34th World Medical Assembly at Lisbon. The preamble states that while a physician should always act according to his/her conscience, and always in the best interests of the patient, equal effort must be made to guarantee patients autonomy and justice. This Declaration represents some of the principal rights of the patient that the medical profession endorses and promotes. Available at http://www.wma.net/en/30publications/10policies/l4/ (accessed 25 April 2015). (The Declaration of Lisbon).

[82] See CESCR General Comment No 14 para 12.

health conditions and the right to access their medical records. The healthcare providers who are motivated by financial gains are not always disposed to providing information to the patients on reasonable treatment options, the available alternatives and the likely benefits and risks of proposed treatment and non-treatment. In *KH and Others v Slovakia*[83] the applicants who could not conceive after consultations with the gynecologists hospitals suspected that they were sterilised and demanded for their medical records. The hospitals refused to release their medical records to their authorised legal representatives or to allow them to obtain copy of the documents. The European Court held that the hospitals refusal amounted to a violation of the rights of the women to information and access to justice.

Similarly, in *Roche v United Kingdom*[84] the defence establishment had conducted a research into chemical weapons for the UK's armed forces, including tests of gases on humans and animals. The applicant, a serviceman, complained that he was not given adequate information about the tests performed on him. The Court found that the State has not fulfilled the positive obligation to provide an effective and accessible procedure enabling the applicant to have access to all relevant and appropriate information that would allow him to assess any risk to which he had been exposed during his participation in the tests.

The medical field is yet to agree on the extent of information a physician is required to disclose to the patient. There is however a firm understanding that the consent of a patient is required before administering treatment, and that consent cannot be real without adequate information. Pattinson observed that it would be impractical for the law to require a doctor to disclose all the known risks of a procedure to all patients. A patient is not usually in a position to understand or absorb all that information, or resolve conflicts in professional opinion. Conversely, a patient who knows nothing about a procedure cannot be said to have

---

[83] App. No. 32881/04 (ECtHR) (April 28, 2009).
[84] App. No. 32555/96 (ECtHR) (October19, 2005).

consented to it. The law requires something between these two extremes.[85] Brazier suggests that within a reformulated fiduciary relationship "the doctor's duty would be to make available to the patient that information that it seems likely that individual patients would need to make an informed choice on treatment."[86]

The judiciary has descended into the arena of this debate. In *Chatterton v Garson*[87] Bristow J held that once the patient is informed in broad terms of the nature of the procedure which is intended, and gives his consent, that consent is real. In *Sideway v Bethlem Royal Hospital*[88] the House of Lords held that a doctor need only disclose such information as would be disclosed by a reasonable body of medical opinion. The court supports the view earlier expressed by McNair J while addressing the jury in *Bolam v Friern Hospital Management Committee*[89] where the judge stated that "[a] doctor is not guilty of negligence if he has acted in accordance with a practice accepted as proper by a responsible body of medical man skilled in that particular art."

The views of the courts in these cases promote the concept of medical paternalism which prefers the opinion of the physician on what is best for the patient. This judicial approach has however witnessed some modifications in the more recent cases. In *Pearce v United Bristol Healthcare NHS Trust*[90] Lord Woolf observed, in a majority decision of the European Community Court, that "if there is a significant risk which would affect the judgment of a reasonable patient, then in the normal course it is the responsibility of a doctor to inform the patient of that significant risk." This position was approved by the House of Lords in *Chester v Afshar*[91] where Lord Steyn stated that "[i]n modern law medical paternalism no longer rules and a patient has a *prima facie* right to be

---

[85] Shaun D. Pattinson, *Medical Law and Ethics* 2ⁿᵈ ed, (London: Sweet &Maxwell Ltd, 2009) 119.

[86] Margaret Brazier, *Medicine, Patient and the Law* 3ʳᵈ ed (London: Penguin, 2003) 110 referred in Pattinson ibid, p 123.

[87] [1981] 1 QB 432 at 443.

[88] [1985] AC 871.

[89] [1957] 2 All ER 118 at 122.

[90] [1999] PIQR 35 at 49.

[91] [2004] UKHL 41 para 16.

informed by a surgeon of a small, but well established, risk of serious injury as a result of surgery."

The preferred position, it is submitted, is that the physician should disclose to the patient, especially when the patient is conscious and is of age, all the medical procedure that would enable the patient to give an informed consent to a particular medical procedure. A physician who assumes a paternalistic position in deciding what is good for the patient could be exposing himself/herself to a legal action that might arise from such conduct. It would seem, however, that in exceptional circumstances such as where the health of an infant is involved, the courts may not hesitate to approve a decision considered by the physician as being in the best interests of the patient. The Supreme Court of Nigeria demonstrated that disposition in *Esabunor & Anor v. Faweya & Ors*[92] where the court in approving blood transfusion to the child against the declining of consent by the parent, held that it could have amounted to a great injustice to the child if the Court had stood by and watched the child being denied of basic treatment to save his life on the basis of the religious conviction of his parent. The child probably would not be alive today. In a life threatening situation, such as the 1st Appellant was in as a child, the consideration to save his life by application of blood transfusion greatly outweighs whatever religious beliefs one may hold, especially where the patient is a child.

A decision such as the above provides a useful guide in defining the relationship between the health workers and the children infected either directly or indirectly by the EVD, especially in the DRC. A report by Unicef indicates that children represent a high proportion among the confirmed cases of Ebola. About 30 per cent of confirmed cases are children. More than 2100 children have been orphaned or left unaccompanied as a result of the Ebola outbreak. This figure includes children who have lost one or both parents, or primary caregivers to Ebola, as well as those who have been left unaccompanied while their parents are isolated in Ebola treatment centers. The impact of the disease on children

---

[92] [2019] LPELR-46961(SC) at 36-38.

is not limited to the children that have been or are infected by the disease. It impacts their families and communities when children lose their parents, care-givers and teachers. Also, the outbreak makes basic services such as health care and education much harder to access.[93] The paternalistic approach by the health care providers would most appropriately address the needs of the children in the prevailing circumstances. There would be no basis for an argument on the requirement of consent of a non-existant or unavailable parent to provide medical assistance to a child whose health and invariably life is at a high risk of extermination by a disease that has posed such daunting challenge to humanity.

However, that argument cannot prevail in all cases. There are reports showing that EVD victims were usually quarantined at specific locations and with little or no medical care. Some were reported to have escaped or attempted to escape from such confinements.[94] These suggest that the victims were neither informed nor consented to such confinements. Such conducts constitute acts of infringement on the right of the victims to be informed by the healthcare providers and the state. The real concern on the need to mitigate the human rights implications of such confinement materially influenced the development of the CUBE which is presently in use in the DRC. The CUBE is a Biosecure Emergency Care Unit, for outbreaks of highly infectious diseases, which allows health care workers to monitor the patient, check their vital signs and administer certain treatments and care from the exterior, without having to wear full Personal Protective Equipment (PPE) suits.[95] This is unlike a typical Ebola treatment unit which isolates patients in rooms where doctors and nurses only briefly enter wearing "PPEs" or heavy protective gear. The CUBE allows doctors more hands-on care and allows family members to visit the patients.

---

[93] Unicef, 'Ebola Outbreak in the Democratic Republic of Congo' available at https://www.unicef.org/wca/ebola-outbreak-democratic-republic-congo (accessed 10 July 2019).

[94] Ebola Patients Keep Escaping Liberian Hospitals available at www.businessinsider.com/r-ebola-outbreak-stirs-anger-in-fragile-liberia (accessed 25 April 2015); See also Ebola Victim in Sierra Leone Escapes from Hospital available at www.bellanaija.com/.../ebola-victim-in-sierra-leone-escapes-from-hospit (accessed 30 April 2017).

[95] The World staff, 'In DR Congo, health workers pioneer new Ebola isolation 'CUBE' available at https://www.pri.org/stories/2019-07-09/dr-congo-health-workers-pioneer-new-ebola-isolation-cube (accessed on 10 July 2019).

Family members can also safely talk with and see the patient throughout the course of treatment as the CUBE has transparent walls. Dr Richard Kojan, president of the Alliance for International Medical Action (ALIMA), who works at the treatment center with the CUBEs explained the importance of the CUBE where he stated that: "One of the good things in this outbreak [in the DRC] is that our design facilitates contact between the patient and their family, between the family and us, the health workers. So, the family, they are there. They see their children and we discuss with them, we explain to them the situation, the evaluation of their children. They sit around the CUBE, they are near their children all the time they need."[96] This innovative approach to treatment and interactions with the infected persons instill confidence in the patients and enhance the recovery process, unlike the cases of total isolation where patients would conceiveable regard themselves as rejected by the society with death appearing more desirable than life.

5.3. Ebola Victims and Right to Privacy and Confidentiality

The word 'privacy' evolved from the Latin word '*privatus*' meaning; apart from the state; peculiar to one's self; of or belonging to an individual; private'.[97] In the simplest sense, 'right to privacy' connotes the right to control information about oneself.[98] The right to privacy is the epicentre of all human freedoms and rights. It has become so important that it is a recurring provision in various international human rights instruments and constitutions of different countries.[99]

The ICCPR contains provisions recognizing the right to privacy in article 17(1) which provides that "[n]o one shall be subjected to arbitrary or unlawful interference with his privacy, family, home or correspondence, nor to unlawful attacks on his honour and reputation". Similarly, the CRC

---

[96] Ibid.

[97] VJ Samar, *The Right to Privacy, Gays, Lesbians and the Constitution* (Philadelphia, Temple University Press, 1991)19.

[98] JHF Shattuck, *Rights of Privacy* (USA, National Textbook Co 1977) 13.

[99] Odunsi & Nwafor op cit p. 251.

provides in article 16(1) that "[n]o child shall be subjected to arbitrary or unlawful interference with his or her privacy, family, home or correspondence, nor to unlawful attacks on his or her honour and reputation".

At the national level, the Nigerian National Health Act of 2014 provides in section 26 (1) that all information concerning a user, including information relating to his or her health status, treatment or stay in a health establishment is confidential. The constitutions of Nigeria, Sierra Leone, Guinea, Liberia and DRC all embody provisions on the protection of the right to privacy. Section 37 of the Nigerian Constitution, for instance, provides that the privacy of citizens, their homes, correspondence, telephone conversations and telegraphic communications is hereby guaranteed and protected.[100] The courts have accommodated various situations within the ambit of privacy. In *Mark v Seattle Times*[101] the Supreme of Washington held that the protectable interest in privacy generally involves at least four distinct types of invasion, namely: intrusion, disclosure, false light and appropriation. In relation to medical jurisprudence, the right of a woman to have an abortion has been upheld as a right to privacy.[102] Similarly, the right to privacy has been adopted to justify the right of a minor to receive contraceptive.[103] In *Georgina Ahamefula v Imperial Medical Centre*[104] the High Court in Nigeria held that an unauthorized testing of the plaintiff's HIV status without consent was unlawful being an interference with an individual's privacy and encroachment on bodily integrity.

In the realm of medical law and ethics, the right to privacy translates to medical confidentiality. Confidentiality is one of the core tenets of medical practice. In the daily exercise of their functions, the physician receives private communications from the patient which the physician is bound to

---

[100] See similar provisions under s 22 of the Sierra Leonean Constitution, arts 12 and 16 of Guinean and Liberian Constitutions respectively, and art 31 of the Constitution of the DRC.
[101] 96 WN 2nd 473, 635 P. 2d 1081 (1981).
[102] *Roe v Wade* 410 US 113; *R v Morgentaler* [1988] 1 SCR 30.
[103] *Carey v Population Services International* 431 US 678 (1977).
[104] Suit No.ID/16272000 (September 27, 2012). (Lagos State High Court).

keep secret and in confidence.[105] The need for medical confidentiality is recognised by various international instruments and medical ethics. The UN Committee on Economic, Social and Cultural Rights (CESCR) General Comment No 14 recognises that the need for the public to be informed should not impair the right to have personal health data treated with confidentiality.[106] In other words, the patient's right to the preservation of health-related information supersedes the public interest in that context. The World Medical Association Declaration of Lisbon on the Right of the Patient (Declaration of Lisbon) states that "[a]ll identifiable information about a patient's health status, medical condition, diagnosis, prognosis   and treatment and all other information of a personal kind must be kept confidential even after death."[107] The Convention on Human Rights and Biomedicine provides in article 10 that everyone has the right to respect for private life in relation to information about his or her health.

There are good reasons for insisting that information given to the physician by the patient be preserved. Firstly, is the right of the patient to medical autonomy. Secondly are the likely consequences which unguarded disclosure of information may have on the patient. In cases of information which may expose the patient to stigmatization and discrimination, the patient could be treated as an outcast in the society.[108] In *Jansen Van Vuuren v Kruger*[109] Harms AJA observed that:

> There are in the case of [highly infectious disease] special circumstances justifying the protection of confidentiality. By the very nature of the disease, it is essential that persons who are at risk should seek medical advice or treatment. Disclosure of the condition has serious personal and social consequences for the patient. He is often isolated or rejected by others which may lead to increased anxiety, depression and psychological conditions.

---

[105] See Odunsi & Nwafor op cit p. 253.
[106] General comment No 14 para 12.
[107] Declaration of Lisbon para 8.
[108] See Odunsi & Nwafor op cit pp. 253-254.
[109] 1993 (4) SA 842 (AD) at 31.

Thirdly is the need to afford the patient an opportunity to give health information freely and confidently to the physician. This is recognised by the British Medical Association guidance where it is stated as follows:

> Confidentiality is an essential requirement for the preservation of trust between patients and health professionals.... Patients should be able to expect that information about their health which they give in confidence will be kept confidential unless there is a compelling reason why it should not. There is also a strong public interest in maintaining confidentiality so that individuals will be encouraged to seek appropriate treatment and share information relevant to it.[110]

Fourthly is the preservation of public interests which is assured when a patient seeks medical solution to ailments. This was recognised in *X v Y*[111] where Rose J said:

> In the long run, preservation of confidentiality is the only way of securing public health; otherwise doctors will be discredited as a source of education, for future individual patients will not come forward if doctors are going to squeal on them. Consequently, confidentiality is vital to secure public as well as private health, for unless those infected come forward they cannot be counselled and self-treatment does not provide the best care.

Patient's privacy and confidentiality are often infringed by healthcare providers. Acts of infringement include; (i) allowing access to patient's medical information to other hospital staff, including those not involved in the individual patient's care. A patient's health information should not be accessible to every healthcare giver in a healthcare center. A nurse whose

---

[110] See British Medical Association, "Confidentiality and disclosure of health information tool kit" available at bma.org.uk/-/media/files/pdfs/.../ethics/confidentialitytoolkit_full.pdf (accessed 26 April 2015). *See also South African Medical and Dental Council Rule 16.*

[111] [1988] 2 All ER 648 (QBD) 653 para a-b. See also *Hague v Williams* [1962] 181 Atlantic Reporter 2d 345 at 349 where the court held that "[a] patient should be entitled freely to disclose his symptoms and condition to his doctor in order to receive proper treatment without fear that those facts may become public property. Only thus can the purpose of the relationship be fulfilled."

role is to vaccinate a patient, should not ordinarily have access to that patient's private mental health records as the information is not relevant to the treatment being provided at that moment. (ii) Conducting medical examinations under public conditions. Privacy and confidentiality are crucial for patients seeking diagnosis and treatment of illnesses that attracts stigma, such as EVD.[112] The testing of persons for Ebola virus at public places and in the public glare infringes on patient's confidentiality.

The right to confidentiality of health information should not interfere with the right to access of private health information. While a holder of private health information is prohibited from sharing that information with anyone who is not essential to providing health care to the patient, the holder must grant the patient access to their private health information upon the patient's request. Patients have the right to access their own health information and to control how such information is shared with other persons. The right to confidentiality of private health information, as well as the right to accessibility of private health information are patient's rights and should be respected by the healthcare providers.[113] In *Jansen Van Vuuren v Kruger* [114] a medical practitioner had disclosed the HIV status of his patient at a golf game after an explicit request by the patient to keep the information confidential to other health practitioners. The patient instituted proceedings claiming that the medical practitioner owed him a duty of confidentiality in relation to any information relating to the plaintiff/patient's medical conditions. The patient argued that he had suffered an invasion of his privacy and had been injured in his rights of privacy. The medical practitioner contended that he had a social and moral duty to make the disclosure to the other health practitioners and that they had a reciprocal social and moral right to receive the information and apply due diligence when again dealing with or treating the plaintiff. Harms AJA held that AIDS is a dangerous condition, but that on its own does not detract from the right of privacy of the afflicted person, especially if that

---

[112] 'Health and Human Rights Resource Guide' Harvard School of Public Heath: Harvard University available at http://hhrguide.org/wp-content/uploads/sites/25/2014/03/ HHRRG-master.pdf (accessed 12 January 2018).
[113] Ibid.
[114] 1993 (4) SA 842 (AD).

right is founded in the doctor-patient relationship. A patient has the right to expect due compliance by the practitioner with his professional ethical standards: in this case the expectation was even more pronounced because of the express undertaking by the first defendant. The practitioners were not at risk and there was no reason to assume that they had to fear a prospective exposure. In consequence the judge concluded that the communication to the practitioners was unreasonable and therefore unjustified and wrongful. The court further emphasised that the duty of medical practitioners to respect the confidence of their patients is not merely an ethical duty but also a legal duty recognised by South African common law. In *MS v Sweden*[115] the Court held that the protection of personal data, particularly medical data, is of fundamental importance to a person's enjoyment of his or her right to respect of private and family life. It was further held that respecting the confidentiality of health data is vital and crucial not only to the privacy of the patient but also to preserve his or her confidence in the medical profession and in the health services in general. In *Z v Finland*[116] the court emphasised that "[w]ithout such protection, those in need of medical assistance may be deterred from revealing such information of a personal and intimate nature as may be necessary in order to receive appropriate treatment and, even from seeking such assistance, thereby endangering their own health and, in the case of transmissible diseases, that of the community."

The non-observance of privacy and confidentiality in the screening and treatment of Ebola victims is one of the reasons that have driven infected persons underground and hence contributed to the spread of the disease in the affected countries.[117] Screening is often done in public. Those who manifest symptoms of the disease are separated from others in the public glare.[118] The emaciated bodies of the victims are often shown on public television where they are isolated with very little medical attention and

---

[115] App. No. 20837/92 (ECtHR) (August 27, 1997).

[116] App. No. 22009/93 (ECtHR) (February 25, 1997) para 95.

[117] 'Guinea residents refusing Ebola treatment' available at http://www.aljazeera.com/news/africa/2014/09/guinea-residents-refusing-ebola-treatment-201492751955453636.html (assessed 16 May 2015).

[118] Guinea: screening for Ebola at Conakry International Airport available at http://www.who.int/features/2014/airport-exit-screening/en/ (accessed 15 May 2018).

awaiting their eventual death. Even the dead are not spared this unnecessary exposure as men in medical protective gear are often shown conveying such bodies to the designated burial places. These conducts have adverse impacts on the families of such victims who are usually avoided as the disease is said to be transmissible by body contacts. There is every cause to believe that unless persons infected with the EVD are assured of their privacy and confidentiality, the victims will not be willing to voluntarily submit themselves for testing and treatment.

5.4. Ebola Victims and Right to Non-Discrimination

The UN Committee on Economic, Social, and Cultural Rights defines discrimination as any "distinction, exclusion, restriction or preference or other differential treatment that is directly or indirectly based on the prohibited grounds of discrimination and which has the intention or effect of nullifying or impairing the recognition, enjoyment or exercise, on an equal footing, of covenant rights".[119] A person is discriminated against when he is treated differently from others and in a manner that undermines his humanness. Discrimination is often associated with stigma. The quest by law to prevent discrimination is necessitated by the stigma attached to people who are given inhuman or degrading treatment. Stigma is a powerful and discrediting social label that radically changes the way individuals view themselves and are viewed as persons.[120] People who are stigmatized are usually treated as outcast or shameful for some reasons and as a result are shunned, avoided, discredited, rejected, restrained or penalized. Reports have shown that the fear and stigma surrounding EVD infection results in people not seeking expert medical advice until they manifest the symptoms of the disease. The fear of being stigmatized or

---

[119] Committee on Economic, Social and Cultural Rights General Comment No 20, Non-discrimination in Economic, Social and Cultural Rights (art 2, para 2) U.N Doc. E/C.12/GC/20 (2009).

[120] S. Iwuagwu, E. Durojaiye et al, *Human Rights and HIV/AIDS: Experience of people living with HIV/AIDS in Nigeria* (Nigeria: CRH Publication 2001) p. 6.

isolated may also cause people to conceal their illness.[121] Reports suggest that the panic surrounding the Ebola virus pandemic affected healthcare providers and led to discrimination against patients suspected of being infected.[122] The social hardship suffered by people who are stigmatized is one of the reasons for the provision of the right to non-discrimination.

It should be emphasised that acts of discrimination offend international and national human rights instruments. The ICCPR provides in article 26 that: "All persons are equal before the law and are entitled without any discrimination to the equal protection of the law. In this respect, the law shall prohibit any discrimination and guarantee to all persons equal and effective protection against discrimination on any ground such as race, colour, sex, language, religion, political or other opinion, national or social origin, property, birth or other status". In the same vein, article 2(2) of the ICESCR provides that the States Parties to the Covenant undertake "to guarantee that the rights enunciated in the present Covenant will be exercised without discrimination of any kind as to race, colour, sex, language, religion, political or other opinion, national or social origin, property, birth or other status". Similarly, article 2 of the African Charter provides that: "Every individual shall be entitled to the enjoyment of the rights and freedoms recognized and guaranteed in the present Charter without distinction of any kind such as race, ethnic group, color, sex, language, religion, political or any other opinion, national and social origin, fortune, birth or other status".

The phrase 'or other status' has been interpreted by the CESCR General Comment No 20 to include health status. "Health status refers to a person's physical or mental health".[123] The CESCR enjoins the states parties to ensure that a person's actual or perceived health status is not a barrier to realizing the rights under the Covenant.[124] The Constitutions of

---

[121] International Federation of Red Cross and Red Crescent 'Battling fear and stigma over Ebola in West Africa-IFRC' available at http://www.ifrc.org/en/news-and-media/news-stories/africa/guinea/battling-fear-and-stigm (accessed 22 September 2018).

[122] Ebola hysteria causes discrimination against patients-health department 'available at http://mg.co.za/article/2014-o8-30-ebola-hysteria-causing-discrimination-against-patients (accessed 29 September 2018).

[123] General Comment No. 20 para 33.

[124] Ibid.

the affected African nations respectively embody provisions against discrimination.[125]

It is observed in the UN General Comment that the protection of public health is often cited by states as a basis for restricting human rights in the context of a person's health status. However, many such restrictions are discriminatory, for example, when HIV status is used as the basis for differential treatment with regard to access to education, employment, healthcare, travel, social security, housing and asylum.[126] The courts in South Africa have similarly held that discrimination on ground of health status (especially on HIV status) is unlawful. In *Hoffmann v South African Airways*[127] Ngcobo J said:

> Society has responded to [the plight of those living with HIV] with intense prejudice. They have been subjected to systemic disadvantage and discrimination. They have been stigmatized and marginalised…. Society's response to them has forced many of them not to reveal their HIV status for fear of prejudice. This in turn has deprived them of the help they would otherwise have received… any discrimination against them can, to my mind, be interpreted as a fresh instance of stigmatization and I consider this to be an assault on their dignity. The impact of discrimination on HIV positive people is devastating. It denies them the right to earn a living. For this reason, they enjoy special protection in our law.

Although the medically established mode of transmission of HIV is not the same as Ebola, the Ebola patients should not be discriminated against, especially in the provision of healthcare, simply on account of their health condition. What is needed is the balancing of the interests of the patient with those of the wider society as stated by the Indian court in *MX of Bombay Indian Inhabitant v M/s ZY and another*[128] as follows:

---

[125] See ss 42 and 27 of the Nigerian and Sierra Leonean Constitutions respectively, as well as arts 18, 8 and 13 of the Liberian, Guinean and DRC Constitutions respectively.

[126] General Comment No 20 para 33.

[127] 2001 (1) SA 1 (CC) para 28. See also *Allpass v Mooikloof Estates (Pty) Ltd t/a Mooikloof Equestrain Centre* 2011 (2) SA 638 (LC).

[128] AIR 1997 (Bombay) 406 at 431.

Taking into consideration the widespread and present threat of this disease [HIV/AIDS] in the world in general ... the State cannot be permitted to condemn the victims ...many of whom may be truly unfortunate, to certain ... death. It is not in the general public interest and is impermissible under the Constitution. The interests of the [victims] ... and the interests of the society will have to be balanced in such a case.

In *Hamel v Malaxos*[129] it was held that a physician must not deny treatment to patients because their medical condition may put the physician at risk. If a patient poses a risk to the physician's health or safety, the physician should take all available steps to minimise the risk before providing treatment or making other suitable alternative arrangement for providing treatment.

This decision justifies the wearing of protective gear by healthcare providers attending to the EVD patients. Though there is always the need for the protection of the wider society as suggested by the above decisions, there is however no justification for abandoning such patients or confining them in their homes or in designated healthcare centres without medical facilities as was the case in some of the affected countries at the initial stages of the outbreak of the EVD.

5.5. Ebola Victims and Freedom from Torture

Article 7 of the ICCPR provides that no one shall be subjected to torture or to cruel, inhuman or degrading treatment or punishment. In particular, no one shall be subjected without his free consent to medical or scientific experimentation. Similarly, article 5 of the Universal Declaration provides that no one shall be subjected to torture or to cruel, inhuman or degrading treatment or punishment. At the regional level, the African Women's Protocol in article 4(1) prohibits all forms of exploitation, cruel,

---

[129] 25, Nov. 1993, No:730-32-oo37929, small claims court Joliette (Unreported) available at www.anilaggrawal.com>...>Reviews>TechnicalBooks (accessed 11 February 2015); See also Stanislaw Frankowski, *Legal responses to AIDS in comparative perspective* 1ˢᵗ ed (Netherlands: Imprint of Brill Academic Publishers, 1998) p87.

inhuman or degrading punishment and treatment. There are also provisions in the constitutions of the African nations in similar terms as the above international instruments.[130]

In *Keenan v United Kingdom*[131] the European Court of Human Rights stated that ill-treatment must attain a minimum level of severity if it is to fall within the scope of Article 3.[132] The assessment of this minimum requirement is relative; it depends on all the circumstances of the case, such as the duration of the treatment, its physical and/or mental effects and, in some cases, the sex, age and state of health of the victim.

The denial of healthcare to incarcerated persons even on account of commission of crime has been held by the courts to amount to torture, cruel and inhuman treatment. This was the position unanimously adopted by the European Court in *Hurtado v. Switzerland*[133] where the court held that the state's failure to provide timeous medical treatment to the detained applicant was an act of inhuman and degrading treatment.

Such denial of medical care could also constitute an infringement on the right to healthcare of the incarcerated person. In *Festus Odaife & Others v Attorney General of the Federation and Others*[134] the applicants who were detainees at the maximum security prison in Lagos, Nigeria contracted HIV while in detention and were denied the right to treatment by the prison officials. In an action to enforce their fundamental rights under the Nigerian Constitution and the African Charter, the court held that the denial of treatment to the four prisoners violated section 8 of the Nigerian Prison Act of 1972 and article 16 of the African Charter. The trial judge emphasised the obligation of the government in the enforcement of the socio-economic rights, especially the right to health, under the African Charter as follows:

---

[130] See ss 34(1)(a) and 20 of Nigerian and Sierra Leonean Constitutions respectively, arts 6, 21(e) and 16 of the Guinean, Liberian and DRC Constitutions respectively.

[131] App. No. 27229/95 (ECtHR) (April3, 2001).

[132] Article 3 of the European Convention on Human Rights similarly prohibits torture, inhuman and degrading treatment.

[133] App. No. 17549/90 (ECtHR) (January 28, 1994).

[134] (2004) AHRLR 205 (NgHC2004).

The government of this country has incorporated the African Charter on Human and Peoples' Rights Cap 10 as part of the law of the country....The Charter entrenched the socio-economic rights of a person. The Court is enjoined to ensure the observation of these rights. A dispute concerning socio-economic rights such as the right to medical attention requires the Court to evaluate state policy and give judgment consistent with the Constitution. I therefore appreciate the fact that the economic cost of embarking on medical provision is quite high. However, the statutes have to be complied with and the state has a responsibility to all the inmates in prison, regardless of the offence involved, as in the instant case where...the applicants... have been in custody for not less than two years suffering from an illness. They cannot help themselves even if they wanted to because they are detained and cannot consult their doctor. I therefore...order the authorities...[to] relocate the applicants after the precondition has been complied with, to a hospital in accordance with section 8 of the Prison Act.[135]

The African Regional Courts have adopted a similar stance in comparable circumstances. The decision of the African Commission on Human and Peoples' Rights in *International Pen and Others (on behalf of Ken Saro Wiwa) v Nigeria*[136] lends credence to this assertion. In that case, Saro Wiwa, a writer and environmental rights activist, together with eight others, were sentenced to death for their social crusade activities in Ogoni land in the Niger Delta region of Nigeria. While in detention awaiting execution, Saro Wiwa's health deteriorated to the point that he required medical attention. The Nigerian government denied him access to treatment in spite of the prison doctor's recommendations. The African Commission held that Saro Wiwa's right to health under article 16 of the African Charter was violated by the Nigerian government. In arriving at this decision, the Commission stated as follows:

The responsibility of the government is heightened in cases where an individual is in its custody and therefore someone whose integrity and well-being are completely dependent on the actions of the authorities.

[135] Ibid paras 37-39.
[136] (2000) AHLR 212(ACHPR 1998).

The state has a direct responsibility in this case. Despite requests for hospital treatment made by a qualified prison doctor, these were denied to Ken Saro Wiwa, causing his health to suffer to the point his life was endangered.... This is a violation of article 16.[137]

Similarly, in *Purohit & More v The Gambia*[138] the Commission emphasised that the:

> Enjoyment of the human rights to health as it is widely known is vital to all aspects of a person's life and well-being, and is crucial to the realization of all the other fundamental human rights and freedoms. This right includes the right to health facilities, access to goods and services to be guaranteed to all without discrimination of any kind.

The victims of Ebola were reportedly confined in their homes or at designated health centers without quality care, functioning water supply and no air conditioning facilities. The families of the patients were responsible their medical and sanitary needs and general upkeep.[139] This is against the legal injunction as espoused by the European court in *Keenan v. United Kingdom*[140] to the effect that persons in custody are in a vulnerable position and that the authorities are under a duty to protect them.

There is therefore an enhanced responsibility on the governments of the affected countries to ensure that the health need of the victims of EVD who are quarantined or confined at designated centres are fully addressed. Failures on the part of the government to provide medical care for EVD patients in such confinements constitute torture and cruel, inhuman, and

---

[137] Article 16 of the ACHPR provides that "(1) Every individual shall have the right to enjoy the best attainable state of physical and mental health. (2) State parties to the present Charter shall take the necessary measures to protect the health of their people and to ensure that they receive medical attention when they are sick."

[138] (2003) AHLRA 96 at 108.

[139] Ebola Patients Abandoned, Health Team Down Tools- Health- Nairaland' available at http://www.nairaland.com/1862229/ebola-patients-abondoned-health-team (accessed 9 September 2014); See also 'Nigeria Hasn't Given Priority To Ebola Treatment, Abandons Nano Silver Treatment' available at http://www.nursingworldnigeria.com/2014/08/nigeria-hasn-rsquo-t-given-priority-to-e (accessed 9 September 2014).

[140] App. No. 27229/95 (ECtHR) (April 3, 2000).

degrading treatment, and also an infringement of the right to healthcare of such victims.

The insistence on the observation of the law and respecting the rights of the victims of the EVD must not however overlook the major constraints which are attendant to the enforcement of such rights from a pragmatic perspective. Most of the Africa nations that were affected by the outbreak of the disease are among the poorest in the world's economic ranking. Some of them are also reeling under the pang of civil strife and political instability which restrict access to certain parts of the country for security and safety reasons. The WHO had, for instance, described the effort at containing the ongoing Ebola virus disease (EVD) outbreak in the Democratic Republic of the Congo as a complex and challenging task, though it remains confident that the outbreak can be successfully contained in collaboration with the Ministry of Health (MoH) and partners. The WHO stated that on 16 November 2018, an armed group attacked the United Nations Organization Stabilization Mission in the Democratic Republic of the Congo (MONUSCO) base in the Boikene District, in the city of Beni, close to the UN Ebola response residences. Response operations in Beni were briefly paused but all activities, including vaccination, resumed by 18 November. WHO condemned the attacks on peacekeepers who are integral to the ongoing efforts to manage the EVD outbreak.[141] In a related incidence, Forbes reported that health workers fighting to contain an Ebola outbreak in DRC, the second largest in history, are finding themselves under attack as more than 30 armed militia groups vie for control of the region. Treatment centers and health workers have been repeatedly targeted, hampering efforts to contain the virus. In April, World Health Organization (WHO) epidemiologist Dr. Richard Valery Mouzoko Kiboung, 42, was shot and killed during an attack at Butembo University Hospital, where he was chairing a meeting with front-line health workers battling the Ebola virus disease.[142] Such incidences certainly

---

[141] "Ebola virus disease – Democratic Republic of the Congo" available at https://www.who.int/csr/don/22-november-2018-ebola-drc/en/ (accessed 16/12/2018).

[142] Sarah Ferguson, "An Ebola Outbreak Rages in Democratic Republic of Congo" available at https://www.forbes.com/sites/unicefusa/2019/05/28/an-ebola-outbreak-rages-in-democratic-republic-of-congo/#6297ed797665 (accessed 09/07/2019).

militate against effective distribution of aid materials and medical facilities to the affected persons.

Where resources are scarce, the tendency would always be to ensure their maximization to guarantee benefit to the greatest number of people in the country. Such an approach has judicial indenture as in *Soobramony v Minister of Health, KwaZulu-Natal*[143] where the South African Constitutional Court alluded to the need to spread scarce state resources to benefit the majority of those in need and not just an individual or a few individuals in the enforcement of socio-economic rights. This again reflects the balancing of public interests with that of individual which though may erode the insistence on the prioritization of the fundamental rights of victims in a public health emergency, is desirable for attaining a greater public goal. There is nothing wrong with that as the individual also needs a safe community to survive. It must however always be borne in mind that human rights are individual rights as given by law, any derogation from such rights in preference for public interests should as such adhere strictly with the enabling law to accord some measure of legitimacy to the adopted policy.

CONCLUSION

The healthcare providers have legal and ethical duties to address a patient's needs that fall within the healthcare provider's scope of practice. Refusing to do so is not consistent with the ethical principle of beneficence. In the wake of the Ebola outbreak in the African nations, healthcare providers were reported to have shown some reluctance, if not out-rightly refusing, to treat the infected patients. Although the healthcare providers need to stay alive in order to attend to the needs of the patient, there seems to be so much emphasis on self-preservation and welfare of the healthcare providers in the affected countries than the interests of the

---

[143] 1998 (1) SA 765 (CC).

patients. Such conducts negate the essence of the ethics that govern the practice of medicine.

The preservation of the victims' interests and guaranteeing of protection of their rights as protected by law are considered very important in the control of the spread of disease in every public health emergency. Such assurances would enable a free and voluntary revelation of the victim's viral status and acceptance of the available preventive or curative measure as would prevent the spreading of the disease.

Admittedly, there is always the issue of overriding public interests which could justify the curtailment of an individual's rights. Both international and national instruments that provide for the rights of the victim also permit a derogation from such rights for the protection of the overriding public interests. It is however important that necessary protocols be followed where the victim's rights are curtailed. For instance, the disclosure of a victim's confidential information by the healthcare provider must be discreetly done and only in situations where there is an identifiable person(s) who is at risk of being infected and the victim would not volunteer such disclosure or grant consent to the healthcare provider to disclose that information. The state should ensure that those in quarantine are fully informed of the reason for placing restrictions on their movement. Such persons should be provided with adequate medical facilities and other amenities to keep them in good health. A blanket lock down of the entire community without food or water and medical facilities, simply on suspicion of the spread of EVD as reported in some of the affected countries cannot be justified under the existing instruments. Governmental efforts at controlling the spread of disease in every public health emergency should be tailored in such a manner as would be perceived generally as preventive or curative and not as punishment for the victims of the disease.

More importantly, however, is that human rights thrive in an environment where there is peace and traquility. The situation in the DRC is an antithesis of those requirements. The international community cannot afford to stand aloof while the burden of disease that has the capacity to exterminate the entire community is exercabated by armed conflict. A concerted effort is urgently needed to restore peace in the DRC and to create a conduce environment for the effective application of the medical solutions in containing the spread of Ebola and the enforcement of the human rights of the infected persons.

REFERENCES

Are Healthcare Providers Legally Obligated to Treat Ebola Patients? available at http://midlevelu.com/blog/are-healthcare-providers-legally-obligated-treat-ebola-patients (accessed 19 Apria 2015).

Are Healthcare Providers Legally Obligated to Treat Ebola Patients? available at http://www.midlevelu.com/blog/are-healcare-providers-legally-obligated-treat-ebola-patients (accessed 4 February 2015).

Barry, HS; Bonnie, HL. '*Ebola, Culture and Politics: The Anthropology of an Emerging Disease*', (2007), available at http:// books.google.com/books? (accessed 3 September 2017).

Belluz, J. 'Seven reasons why this Ebola epidemic spun out of control' available at https://www.vox.com/2014/9/4/6103039/Seven-reasons-why-this-ebola-virus-outbreak-epidemic-out-of-control (accessed 15/12/2018).

Blake, M. 'Dogs eating corpses of Ebola victims in Liberia' *Mail Online* available at https://www.dailymail.co.uk/news/article-2737684/Dogs-EATING-corpses-Ebola-victims-Liberia-health-teams-pile-bodies-shallow-grave-middle-night-locals-refused-permission-use-land.html (accessed 15 December 2018).

Boseley, S.; Burke, J. *'Terrifying' Ebola epidemic out of control in DRC, say experts'* available at https://www.theguardian.com/world/2019/may/15/ebola-in-the-drc-everything-you-need-to-know (accessed on 10 July 2019).

Brazier, M. *Medicine, Patient and the Law* 3rd ed (London: Penguin, 2003).

British Medical Association, '*Confidentiality and disclosure of health information tool kit'* available at bma.org.uk/-/media/files/pdfs/.../ethics/confidentialitytoolkit_full.pdf (accessed 26 April 2015).

Brown, R. 'The virus detective who discovered Ebola in 1976' *News Magazine, BBC News* available at http://www.bbc.co.uk/news/ magazine-28262541 (accessed 6 September 2017).

Burt, A. *'What is the relationship between human rights and human dignity'* available at www.peterjepson.com/law/CIT2-6%20Burt.pdf (accessed 19 June 2017).

Burt, A. *'What is the relationship between human rights and human dignity'* available at www.peterjepson.com/law/CIT2-6%20Burt.pdf (accessed 12 June 2018).

Centers for Disease Control and Prevention, *'Ebola in Democratic Republic of Congo'* available at https://wwwnc.cdc.gov/travel/notices/ alert/ebola-democratic-republic-of-the-congo (accessed 10 July 2019).

Christopher, McCrudden. 'Human Dignity and Judicial Interpretation of Human Rights' (2008) 19 *Issue 4 European Journal of International Law*, 655-724.

Cohen, J. 'Ebola Vaccine is having a 'major impact' but worries about Congo outbreak grow' available at https://www.sciencemag.org/ news/ 2018/12/ebola-vaccine-having-major-impact-outbreak-may-still-explode-west-africa accessed on 12/12/2018.

Cohen, J; Ezer, T. 'Human Rights in Patients Care: A Theoretical and Practical Framework', (2015), 15(2) *Health and Human Rights*, 7.

Committee on Economic, Social and Cultural Rights General Comment No 20, *Non-discrimination in Economic, Social and Cultural Rights* (art 2, para 2) U.N Doc. E/C.12/GC/20 (2009).

Convention on Human Rights and Biomedicine Oviedo, 4.IV.1997 available at http://conventions.coe.int/Treaty/en/Treaties/Html/164.htm (accessed 25 June 2018).

Cornell, D; Woolman, S; Fuller, S; Brickhill, J; Bishop, M; Dunbar, D. *The Dignity Jurisprudence of the Constitutional Court of South Africa*, Vol I (New York, Fordham University Press, 2013).

Dhai, A; McQuoid- Mason, D. *Bioethics, Human Rights and Health: Law, Principle and Practice* (Cape Town: Juta & Co Ltd, 2011).

Dignity and me – RCN www.rcn.org.uk › ... › *CPD online learning* › *Dignity in health care* (accessed 27 January 2016).

Dignity and me – RCN, available at www.rcn.org.uk › ... › *CPD online learning › Dignity in health care* (accessed 19 July 2017).

'Doctor-patient relationship' available at http://en.wikipedia.org/ wiki/ Doctor%E2%80%93patient_relationship (accessed 14 January 2017).

'DR Congo Ebola Outbreak: Child in Uganda dies of virus' available at https://www.bbc.com/news/world-africa-48603273 (accessed 10 July 2019).

Durojaye, E; Ayankogbe, O. 'A rights- based approach to access to HIV treatment in Nigeria', (2005), 5, *African Human Rights Law Journal*, 289.

'Ebola hysteria causes discrimination against patients-health department' available at http://mg.co.za/article/2014-o8-30-ebola-hysteria-causing-discrimination-against-patients (accessed 29 September 2018).

'Ebola in the DRC: everything you need to know' available at https://www.theguardian.com/world/2019/may/15/ebola-in-the-drc-everything-you-need-to-know (accessed 09/07/2019).

'Ebola Patients Abandoned, Health Team Down Tools- Health' Nairaland available at http://www.nairaland.com/1862229/ebola-patients-abondoned-health-team (accessed 9 September 2014).

'Ebola Patients Abandoned, Health Team Down Tools- Health' Nairaland available at http://www.nairaland.com/1862229/ebola-patients-abondoned-health-team (accessed 9 September 2014).

'Ebola Patients Abandoned, Health Team Down Tools- Health' *Nairaland* available at http://www.nairaland.com/1862229/ebola-patients-abondoned-health-team (accessed 9 September 2014).

'Ebola Patients Abandoned, Health Team Down Tools- Health' Nairaland available at http://www.nairaland.com/1862229/ebola-patients-abondoned-health-team (accessed 19 September 2018).

'Ebola Patients Keep Escaping Liberian Hospitals' available at www.businessinsider.com/r-ebola-outbreak-stirs-anger-in-fragile-liberia (accessed 30 April 2017).

'Ebola Victim in Sierra Leone Escapes from Hospital' available at www.bellanaija.com/.../ebola-victim-in-sierra-leone-escapes-from-hospit (accessed 30 April 2017).

'Ebola virus definition- Infectious Disease Center: Information on Infection' *Medicine Net.com* available at http://www.medters.com/script/main/art.asp?articlekey=6518.

'Ebola virus disease – Democratic Republic of the Congo' available at https://www.who.int/csr/don/22-november-2018-ebola-drc/en/ (accessed 16 December 2018).

'Ebola Virus Disease' available at http://en.wikipedia.org/ wiki/ Ebola_virus_disease (accessed 3 September 2014).

'Ebola Virus disease' available at http://en.wikipedia.org/wiki/ Ebola_virus_disease (accessed 3 September 2016).

'Ebola Virus disease' available at http://en.wikipedia.org/wiki/ Ebola_virus_disease (accessed 9 September 2017).

'Ebola Virus disease' available at http://www.who.int/mediacentre/ factsheets/fs103/en/ (accessed 5 September 2017).

'Ebola Virus disease' available at http://www.who.int/mediacentre/ factsheets/fs103/en/ (accessed 5 September 2014).

'Ebola virus: 9 things to know about the killer disease-CNN.com August 25, 2014' available at http://edition.cnn.com/2014/08/07/world/ebola-virus-q-and-a/ (accessed 3 September 2017).

'Ebola Virus' available at https://microbewiki.kenyon.edu/index.php/ Ebola-virus (accessed 3 September 2014);

Elsayed, KA; El-Melegy, OA; El-Zeftawy, AM. 'The Effect of an Educational Intervention on Nurses' Awareness about Patients' Rights in Tanta', (2013), 9(9), *Journal of American Science*, 211.

Emond, RT; Evans, B; ET Bowen, ET; et al. 'A case of Ebola virus infection', (1977), 2, *British Medical Journal*, 541-544.

Ferguson, S. *'An Ebola Outbreak Rages in Democratic Republic of Congo'* available at https://www.forbes.com/sites/unicefusa/2019/05/28/an-ebola-outbreak-rages-in-democratic-republic-of-congo/#6297ed797665 (accessed 09/07/2019).

Forsythe, DP. *Human Rights in International Relations* 2nd ed (New York: Cambridge University Press, 2006), p. 3

Frankowski, S. *Legal responses to AIDS in comparative perspective* 1st ed (Netherlands: Imprint of Brill Academic Publishers, 1998).

Greene, R; Goldschmidt, D. *'Ebola outbreak spreads outside Congo, WHO says'* available at https://edition.cnn.com/2019/06/11/health/ebola-outside-congo-uganda-africa-bn/index.html (accessed on 10 July 2019).

'Guinea residents 'refusing' Ebola treatment' available at http://www.aljazeera.com/news/africa/2014/09/guinea-residents-refusing-ebola-treatment-201492751955453636.html (assessed 16 May 2015).

'Guinea: screening for Ebola at Conakry International Airport' available at http://www.who.int/features/2014/airport-exit-screening/en/ (accessed 15 May 2018).

'Health and Human Rights Resource Guide' Harvard School of Public Health: Harvard University available at http://hhrguide.org/wp-content/uploads/sites/25/2014/03/HHRRG-master.pdf (accessed 12 January 2015).

'Health and Human Rights Resource Guide' Harvard School of Public Heath: Harvard University available at http://hhrguide.org/wp-content/uploads/sites/25/2014/03/HHRRG-master.pdf (accessed 12 January 2018).

'Health and Human Rights' A Resource Guide for the Open Society Institute and Soros Foundations Network June 2007 available at http://kelinkenya.org/wp-content/uploads/2010/10/Health-and-Human-Rights-Resource-Guide-OSI-Equitas.pdf (accessed 25 January 2018).

Healthy Development, The World Bank Strategy for HNP Results Annex L- April 24 2007.

International Federation of Red Cross and Red Crescent *'Battling fear and stigma over Ebola in West Africa-IFRC'* available at http://www.ifrc.org/en/news-and-media/news-stories/africa/guinea/battling-fear-and-stigm (accessed 22 September 2018).

Iwuagwu, S. (ed) *HIV/AIDS and Human Rights: Role of the Judiciary* (Nigeria: CRH Publication, 2001).

Iwuagwu, S; Durojaiye, E; et al., *Human Rights and HIV/AIDS: Experience of people living with HIV/AIDS in Nigeria* (Nigeria: CRH Publication 2001).

Johnson, KM; Webb, PA; Lange, IV; Murphy, FA. *'Isolation and Characterization of a new virus (Ebola virus) causing acute haemorrhagic fever in Zaire'* (1977) 1:569-71, available at http://jid.oxfordjournals.org/content/179/Supplement_1/ix.long.

King, JW. *'Ebola Virus'* (2008) eMedicine, WebMd available at http://www.emedicine.com/MED/topic626.htm (assessed 5 September 2014).

Kuhn, JH; et al. 'proposal for a revised taxonomy of the family Filoviridae: Classification, names of taxa and viruses, and virus abbreviations', (2010), 155 (12), *Archives of Virology*, 2083-130.

Kuhn, JH; et al. 'proposal for a revised taxonomy of the family Filoviridae: Classification, names of taxa and viruses, and virus abbreviations', (2010), 155 (12), *Archives of Virology*, 103.

Landale, J. 'Ebola in DR Congo: Fear and mistrust stalk battle to halt outbreak' available at https://www.bbc.com/news/world-africa-48908993 (accessed on 10 July 2019).

Litman, M. 'Fiduciary law in the hospital context: the prescriptive duty of protective intervention', (2007), 15, *Health Law Journal*, 299.

Ludwig, JO; Burke, W. 'Physician –Patient Relationship' University of Washington School of Medicine, *Ethics in Medicine* available at http://depts..washington.edu/bioethx/topics/physpt.html (accessed 20 July 2018).

Man transports a possible victim of the Ebola virus in a wheelbarrow on Thursday at the Ebola treatment center at Island Hospital in Monrovia, Liberia. (Oct 2, 2014.) Available at http://earthsquare.net/7759 (accessed 15 May 2015).

Medecins Sans Frontieres, *'Ebola Outbreak in DRC: Fighting an epidemic in a conflict zone'* available at https://www.doctorswithoutborders.org/ebola-outbreak-drc (accessed 10 July 2019).

'Nigeria Hasn't Given Priority to Ebola Treatment, Abandons Nano Silver Treatment' available at http://www.nursingworldnigeria.com/2014/08/nigeria-hasn-rsquo-t-given-priority-to-e (accessed 9 September 2016).

'Nigeria Hasn't Given Priority to Ebola Treatment, Abandons Nano Silver Treatment' available at http://www.nursingworldnigeria.com/ 2014/08/ nigeria-hasn-rsquo-t-given-priority-to-e (accessed 19 September 2018).

Nwafor, AO. 'Comparative perspectives on euthanasia in Nigeria and Ethiopia', (2010), 18 (2), *African Journal of International and Comparative Law*, 178.

Nwafor, AO. 'Enforcing Fundamental Rights in Nigerian Courts-Processes and Challenges', (2009), 4, *African Journal of Legal Studies*, 1.

Odunsi, SB; Nwafor, AO. 'Medical Confidentiality: Right of HIV/AIDS Patient and the Third Party Interest', (2006), 16 (2), *Lesotho Law Journal*, 250.

Ojwang, BO; Oguta, EO; Matu, PM. 'Nurses' impoliteness as an impediment to patients' rights in selected Kenyan hospital', (2010), 12 (2), *Health and Human Rights*, 101.

'Opinion 10.01-Fundamental Elements of the patient-Physician Relationship' available at www.ama-assn.org/ama/pub/ physician.../ medical.../opinion1001.page (accessed 4 February 2015).

'Patient care - definition of Patient care' *Medical Dictionary* available at medical-dictionary.thefreedictionary.com/Patient+care (accessed 21 January 2015).

Pattinson, SD. *Medical Law and Ethics* 2nd ed (London: Sweet & Maxwell Ltd, 2009).

Pulia, M. 'Simple Tips to Improve Patients Satisfaction', (2011), 18(1), *American Academy of Emergency Medicine*, 18-19.

Roemer, MI. *National Health Systems of the World*, Vol 1 (New York, Oxford University Press, 1991).

Samar, VJ. *The Right to Privacy, Gays, Lesbians and the Constitution* (Philadelphia, Temple University Press, 1991).

Shah, CS. *'Revival of medical Ethics'* available www.boloji.com/ index.cfm?md=Content&sd=Articles&ArticleID (accessed 4 February 2015).

Shattuck, JHF. *Rights of Privacy* (USA, National Textbook Co, 1977).

'Should doctors "have" to treat Ebola patients? - *AMERICAblog* available at americablog.com/2014/09/doctors-treat-ebola-patients. html (accessed 24 March 2016).

Soucheray, S. *'As Ebola rages on, DRC sees more displaced people'* available at http://www.cidrap.umn.edu/news-perspective/2019/07/ ebola-rages-drc-sees-more-displaced-people (accessed 10 July 2019),

The Declaration of Lisbon 1981 available at http://www.wma.net/en/ 30publications/10policies/l4/ (accessed 25 April 2015).

'The Hippocratic Oath' available at http://www.nlm.nih.gov/hmd/greek/ greek_oath.html (accessed 18 April 2015).

The World staff, In *DR Congo, health workers pioneer new Ebola isolation 'CUBE'* available at https://www.pri.org/stories/2019-07-09/dr-congo-health-workers-pioneer-new-ebola-isolation-cube (accessed on 10 July 2019).

Unicef, *'Ebola Outbreak in the Democratic Republic of Congo'* available at https://www.unicef.org/wca/ebola-outbreak-democratic-republic-congo (accessed 10 July 2019).

Universal Declaration of Human Rights, General Assembly Resolution 217A(111) 10 December 1948.

Universal Declaration of Human Rights, General Assembly Resolution 217A(111) 10 December 1948.

Viljoen, F. *International Human Rights Law in Africa 2nd ed* (United Kingdom: Oxford University Press, 2012).

'West Africa: Respect Rights in Ebola Response| Human Rights Watch' available at http://www.hrw.org/news/2014/09/15/west-africa-respect-rights-ebola-response (accessed 22 September 2017).

'WHO| Patients' rights' available at http://www.who.int/genomics/ public/patientrights/en/ (accessed 23 January 2015).

World Health Organisation Regional Office for the Eastern Mediterranean, *'The Role of Government in Health Development Agenda item 7(a)'* EM/RC53/Tech.Disc.1, July 2006.

World Health Organization Ebola haemorrhagic fever in Sudan (1976) Report of a World Health Organization International Study Team. *Bull WHO*, 1978, (56), 247-270 available at http://whqlibdoc.whoint/

bulletin/1978/Vo156-No2/bulletin_1978_56(2)_247_270.pdf (accessed 5 September 2014).

World Organization 'Ebola haemorrhagic fever in Zaire' 1976. Report of an International Convention. *Bulletin of the World Health Organization*, (1978), 56(2), 271-29, available at http://whqlibdoc.who.int/bulletin/1978/Vol56-No2/bulletin_1978_56(2)_247-270.pdf (accessed 3 September 2016).

Judicial Decisions

Allpass v Mooikloof Estates (Pty) Ltd t/a Mooikloof Equestrain Centre, 2011, (2), SA 638 (LC).

Bolam v Friern Hospital Management Committee, [1957], 2 All ER 118 at 122.

Bristol and West Building Society v Mothew, [1998], Ch 1 at 18A.

Carey v Population Services International, 431 US 678, (1977).

Chatterton v Garson, [1981], 1 QB 432 at 443.

Chester v Afshar, [2004], UKHL 41 para 16.

Dawood and Another v Minister of Home Affairs and Others, Shalabi and Another v Minister of Home Affairs and Others, Thomas and Another v Minister of Home Affairs and Others, 2000, (3) SA 936 (CC) para 35.

Esabunor & Anor v. Faweya & Ors, [2019] LPELR-46961(SC) at 36-38.

Extrasure Travel Insurance Ltd v Scattergood, [2003], 1 BCLC 598 at 617.

Festus Odaife & Others v Attorney General of the Federation and Others, (2004) AHRLR 205 (NgHC2004).

Georgina Ahamefula v Imperial Medical Centre Suit No.ID/16272000 (September 27, 2012). (Lagos State High Court).

Hague v Williams, [1962], 181 Atlantic Reporter 2d 345 at 349

Hamel v Malaxos, 25, Nov. 1993, No: 730-32-oo037929, small claims court Joliette (Unreported) available at www.anilaggrawal.com>...>Reviews>TechnicalBooks (accessed 11 November 2018).

Hoffmann v South African Airways, 2001, (1), SA 1 (CC) para 28.

Hurtado v. Switzerland App. No. 17549/90 (ECtHR) (January 28, 1994).

International Pen and Others (on behalf of Ken Saro Wiwa) v Nigeria, (2000), AHLR 212(ACHPR 1998).

Jansen Van Vuuren v Kruger, 1993 4 SA 842 (AD).

Keenan v United Kingdom App. No. 27229/95 (ECtHR) (April 3, 2001).

KH and Others v Slovakia App. No. 32881/04 (ECtHR) (April 28, 2009).

Le Roux and Others v Dey, 2010 (4) SA 210 (SCA) para 20.

Mark v Seattle Times 96 WN 2nd 473, 635 P. 2d 1081, (1981).

MS v Sweden App. No. 20837/92 (ECtHR) (August 27, 1997).

MX of Bombay Indian Inhabitant v M/s ZY and another AIR, 1997 (Bombay), 406 at 431.

Pearce v United Bristol Healthcare NHS Trust, [1999] PIQR 35 at 49.

Purohit & More v The Gambia, (2003) AHLRA 96 at 108.

Roche v United Kingdom App. No. 32555/96 (ECtHR) (October19, 2005).

Roe v Wade 410 US 113; *R v Morgentaler*, [1988] 1 SCR 30.

S v Makwanyane, 1995 (3) SA 391 (CC) para 328.

Sideway v Bethlem Royal Hospital, [1985] AC 871.

Soobramony v Minister of Health, KwaZulu-Natal, 1998, (1) SA 765 (CC).

Ultraframe (UK) Ltd v Fielding, [2005], EWHC 1638 (Ch) para 1300.

X v Y, [1988] 2 All ER 648 (QBD) 653 para a-b.

Z v Finland App. No. 22009/93 (ECtHR) (February 25, 1997) para 95.

In: Ebola Virus Disease (EVD)   ISBN: 978-1-53616-291-2
Editor: Hilaire Verreau   © 2019 Nova Science Publishers, Inc.

Chapter 4

CONTROL STRATEGIES OF EBOLA VIRUS DISEASE IN BIOINFORMATICS PERSPECTIVE

Eka Gunarti Ningsih
and Usman Sumo Friend Tambunan[*]
Department of Chemistry,
Faculty of Mathematics and Natural Sciences,
Universitas Indonesia, Kampus UI Depok,
West Java, Depok, Indonesia

ABSTRACT

Ebola disease is an acute fever disease that is caused by infection of viruses within the genus *Ebolavirus* such as *Zaire ebolavirus*, *Sudan ebolavirus*, *Bundibugyo ebolavirus*, *Taï Forest ebolavirus*, and *Reston ebolavirus*. Almost all species cause disease in human, except *Reston ebolavirus* which is only known to cause disease in nonhuman primates. Ebola infection in human has similar initial symptoms with influenza or malaria which are marked with pyrexia, sore head, muscle or joint pain, weakness, vomiting, abdomen pain, as well as bleeding. The virus can spread by direct contact from human to human through various bodily

[*] Corresponding Author's Email: usman@ui.ac.id.

fluids such as saliva, blood, stool, semen, breast milk, and tears. Ebola virus proteins comprise of non-structural proteins, nucleoprotein, matrix protein, and glycoproteins. Since its discovery in 1976, Ebola virus has become an epidemic in the African continent. The most extensive Ebola case in history was confirmed at the end of March 2016 with 11,325 deaths in West Africa. Unfortunately, there is no FDA-approved drug to treat this viral infection in human. Drug discovery and development for EVD is a complex process which requires a long time, many resources, and huge capital. Because of that, another approach has to apply in order to reduce all of the necessities. Bioinformatics studies through the Computer-Aided Drug Design (CADD) method can be employed to find the potential drug candidates at the preliminary stage of drug discovery. Our research group has successfully developed drug candidates to treat Ebola by using EBOV protein structure. Most of these drug candidates were obtained from some free online databases and were processed through molecular docking simulation. The drug candidates which was selected must comply with the requirements such as attaching to the binding sites of the protein, have energy binding value lower than standards, and exhibited preferable interaction with the protein. The screening process also involves pharmacokinetics analysis and toxicity prediction by using software to suppress possible failure when evaluated later in the wet laboratory. In this chapter, we describe the successful developed drug candidates from our laboratory to treat Ebola by using EBOV protein structure, such as VP24, VP35, VP40, nucleoprotein, and glycoprotein.

Keywords: Ebola virus disease, bioinformatics, computer-aided drug design, molecular docking

INTRODUCTION

Ebola Virus Disease (EVD) or Ebola Haemorrhagic Fever (EHF) is an acute fever disease in human which often cause death if untreated (World Health Organization 2018). EVD originates from the infection of viruses belonging to the *Filoviridae* family which consist of five species of viruses within the *Ebolavirus* genus namely *Zaire ebolavirus*, *Sudan ebolavirus*, *Bundibugyo ebolavirus*, *Taï Forest ebolavirus*, and *Reston ebolavirus*. Among these species, four viruses cause disease in human, except *Reston ebolavirus* which only infect nonhuman primates (Centers for Disease

Control and Prevention (CDC) 2018). EVD first appeared in 1976 in two near-simultaneous outbreaks in the Democratic Republic of the Congo with 280 deaths of 318 cases and Sudan with 151 deaths of 284 cases. At the end of March 2016, about 28,652 EVD cases were confirmed by WHO with 11,325 deaths, becoming the most extensive West Africa EVD epidemic in history (Bell et al. 2016). Since then, the most recent yet smaller EVD outbreaks reported by CDC were appeared in the Democratic Republic of the Congo from May to July 2017 with 4 deaths of 8 total cases.

Ebola viruses (EBOV) are non-segmented, negative-sense single-stranded RNA containing 18.9-kb RNA genome which is comprised of genes encoding seven structural and one non-structural protein. The proteins are 30 noncoding regions (leader), nucleoprotein (NP), the Virion Protein 24 (VP24), VP30, VP35, VP40, RNA-dependent RNA polymerase (L) and glycoprotein (GP) (Hoenen et al. 2006). Nucleocapsid structures, NP, VP30, VP35, and L are involved in synthesizing virus RNAs while VP24, VP40, and GP are related to the viral membrane (Falasca et al. 2015). The glycoprotein gene encodes the surface GP in two molecular forms, GP1 and GP2, which have an important role for virus entry by binding and fusion of receptor with target cells (Mehedi et al. 2011).

Zaire Ebolavirus has been established as the etiological agent of the epidemic in 2014 (Judson, Prescott, and Munster 2015). In human, EBOV has been identified using Reverse Transcription Polymerase Chain Reaction (RT-PCR) in various bodily fluids such as saliva, blood, stool, semen, breast milk, and tears (Bausch et al. 2007). Another route of EBOV transmission is direct contact with animals, including blood, organs, or prepares meat from infected animals. The animal host of the EBOV is still undiscovered. However, immunoglobulin G (IgG) characteristic for EBOV was detected in fruit bat serum, generally from three different species (*Hypsignathus monstrosus*, *Epomops franqueti*, and *Myonycteris torquata*) which indicate that these animals may be acting as the wild host of EBOV (Leroy et al. 2005). Dogs might be infected with EBOV in the wild environment because of their food, but there are no reports of dog spreading EBOV to people or other animals (Allela et al. 2005).

The symptoms of EBOV infection appear from 2 to 21 days, with an average of 8 to 10 days, after virus contact. EBOV infection in human has similar symptoms with influenza or malaria which are marked with pyrexia, sore head, muscle or joint pain, weakness, vomiting, abdomen pain as well as bleeding (Leligdowicz et al. 2016). These viruses cause disease related to systemic viral replication, fluid and electrolyte losses, abnormal inflammatory responses, immune suppression, and mortality (Malvy et al. 2019). Analyses of Immunohistochemistry (IHC) and electron microscopic from the infected tissues proved that the endothelial cells, hepatocytes, and mononuclear phagocytes are the main targets of EBOV infection (Zaki et al. 1999). Meanwhile, the monocytes, macrophages, dendritic cells, fibroblasts, adrenal cortical cells, and several types of epithelial cells are involved in virus replication (Feldmann and Geisbert 2011). Several mechanisms of immunology are implicated in the pathogenesis of EVD. The infection is able to inhibit of type-I IFNs response and induce massive cytokines or chemokines network by monocytes/macrophages, as well as functional impairment of human dendritic cells and natural killer (NK) cells (Falasca et al. 2015).

There is no FDA-approved drug was reported to treat this viral infection in human, makes EBOV stand of category A in biothreat pathogen that is a paramount public health concern as claimed by the CDC. Residents of rural central Africa are at a high risk of suffering from EVD. The outbreaks are commonly related to limited public health control and insufficient medical preventive measures. Severely ill patients often experience interferes of blood clotting and electrolyte imbalance. Therefore, supportive care when the virus spreads in the human body is the addition of the electrolyte solution via intravenous or oral (Torre, Nicosia, and Cardi 2014). Multiple candidate therapies against EBOV are currently in development and still need a long way before it can be clinically applied (MacNeil and Rollin 2012).

Some pharmaceutical companies have been working to develop drugs against EVD. Tekmira Pharmaceuticals as the example, utilizing small interfering RNAs (siRNAs) complexed with stable nucleic acid-lipid particles (SNALPs) for inhibiting *Zaire ebolavirus* (ZEBOV) polymerase

L protein, known as TKM-Ebola or TKM-130803. According to the research, TKM-Ebola formulation not only protected guinea pigs from lethal ZEBOV infection (T. W. Geisbert et al. 2006), but also completely protected rhesus monkeys against death from EVD (T. W. Geisbert et al. 2010). However, intravenous administration of TKM-Ebola to patients with severe EVD has not improved survival patients in phase 2 clinical trial (Dunning et al. 2016).

AVI-6002 is another drug development on RNA-based therapeutics which used Phosphorodiamidate Morpholino Oligomers (PMO) to improve the stability, function, and bioavailability of anti-sense complex. Treatment with AVI-6002 in mouse, guinea pigs, and rhesus monkeys resulted in high levels of survival after infected of EBOV (Iversen et al. 2012). The early clinical trial was conducted to understand the safety, tolerability, and pharmacokinetics of increasing single doses of AVI-6002 in the subjects. Unfortunately, the results of the study have not been published and further development has been suspended (Bixler, Duplantier, and Bavari 2017).

In other drug development, BCX4430 has demonstrated pronounced efficacy in non-clinical studies about the EBOV infection. Currently, it is still in the process of Phase 1 clinical testing through intramuscular drug administration (Taylor et al. 2016). Moreover, ZMapp, the triple monoclonal antibody cocktail which directed against the surface glycoprotein of EBOV, is still ongoing in phase II clinical trials (Davey et al. 2016). Another example is chloroquine which has been proved able to inhibit EBOV replication. However, chloroquine does not become a treatment strategy for EVD due to the observed unprotective effects in guinea pigs (Dowall et al. 2015).

Besides developing novel drugs, some studies are also conducted to identify different therapeutic agents which have potency against EBOV such as favipiravir. Favipiravir, which also known as T705, is the pyrazinecarboxamide derivative that able to inhibit RNA replication of influenza viruses. T705 is a prospective treatment of severe EBOV disease which was investigated in phase II human clinical trial (Clinical Trials Identifier: NCT02662855). However, no survival was shown to be successful in favipiravir associated with frequent oral dosing during EBOV infection in nonhuman primates (Bixler et al. 2018).

Several specific proteins of EBOV interact with host-cell to encourage the biological activity of the virus such as ATP1A1 and NPC1. Inhibiting ATP1A1 with ouabain can reduce viral replication in human lung cells. However, ouabain might be toxic at high levels and not FDA-approved. Thus, it was not considered as a medical treatment of EVD (García-Dorival et al. 2014). As an alternative, miglustat, clomiphene, and toremifene become the most promising strategy to treat EVD based on their preclinical evidence in living animals. Clomiphene and toremifene are novel Niemann-Pick C1 or NPC1 (host-cell protein) inhibitors while miglustat is usually used for Niemann-Pick C disease treatment (Patterson et al. 2007). However, the oral administration of clomiphene is very low compared to toremifene. Therefore, the combination of toremifene and miglustat will be potential for curing the lethal EBOV infection (Yuan 2015). In addition, in vivo test in non-human primates should be immediately conducted before the human trial stage.

EBOLA CONTROL STRATEGIES

Drug discovery and development is a complex process which requires a long time, many resources, and huge capital (Salazar and Gormley 2017). Moreover, the necessary facilities such as biosafety level four (BSL-4) in EBOV preclinical studies is become a problem because of the limited number of BSL-4 laboratories worldwide. In 2013, Pharmaceutical Research and Manufacturers of America calculated the cost of research and development to produce drugs that the Food and Drug Administration (FDA) approved resulting around $2.6 billion, including the cost of failure (Salazar and Gormley 2017). As the earliest stage in drug development, screening method was used to discover compounds that have activity against a particular disease. At this stage, in silico study is often used to identify drug candidates through drug interaction simulation (Ferreira et al. 2015).

Bioinformatics approach through Computer-Aided Drug Design (CADD) method could be applied to produce more drugs with lower risk in a short period of time. Bioinformatics is the convergence of several scientific disciplines that currently developed rapidly for medical applications. It leads the critical roles for the discovery, assessment, and development of drugs (Teufel et al. 2006). Bioinformatics not only plays in dealing large volumes of data, but also in the application of bioinformatics implements to predict, assess, or interpret clinical and preclinical findings, particularly related to the absorption, distribution, metabolism, excretion, and toxicity of potential drug leads (Wishart 2005).

Generally, CADD technology that was used in our research is Structure-Based Drug Design (SBDD) and Fragment-Based Drug Design (FBDD). SBDD approach is widely used to predict the position of small molecules within the protein that represented in a three-dimensional structure. Moreover, through this approach, the ligand affinity to the target protein can be estimated accurately and efficiently (Wang et al. 2018). SBDD was considered as the proper method for designing a drug that can treat diseases. Before the drug design process, determining the protein structure become the most important thing. Previously, the protein structure was only determined by X-Ray diffraction and NMR methods. For now, the structure can be easily obtained from the Research Collaboratory for Structural Bioinformatics – Protein Data Bank (RCSB PDB) database. If protein structures have not available yet, the 3D structure can be obtained through homology modeling (Huang et al. 2010).

Besides SBDD, Fragment-Based Drug Discovery (FBDD) was also developed to start the lead generation process in drug discovery. For fragment generation, all collected compounds from databases must be screened by using Astex Rule of Three parameters, such as molecular weight less than 300 Da, c Log P less than 3, the number of hydrogen donor less than 3, the number of hydrogen acceptor less than 3, rotatable bond less than 3 and Topological Polar Surface Area (TPSA) less than 60 $Å^2$ (Congreve et al. 2003). Furthermore, chemical fragments which have low molecular weight are initially selected according to their ability to bind to the target of interest (Erlanson, McDowell, and O'Brien 2004). For fragment modification, three main techniques are commonly used such as fragment merging, linking, and growing. Fragment merging is the combining structural parts of fragments that are overlapping into a ligand, using structural information from other fragments, substrates, and ligands known in complexes with proteins. While fragment linking is the joining of two known fragments binding on the non-overlapping site. Different from merging and linking, fragment growing involves a modification process by way of growing the fragments that are known to bind at a single site through chemical synthesis to explore further interactions (Scott et al. 2012).

The molecular docking is a process that occurs when a ligand finds its position in the active sites of the protein after passing a number of movements in its conformation. It purposes of predicting the complex structure of ligand-receptor which involve two interrelated steps. Firstly, predicting the conformation of the ligand based on the position and orientation of pose, then ranking these conformations through a scoring function (Meng et al. 2011). In general, docking is used to conduct virtual screening on large libraries of compounds and proposed a hypothesis about how ligands inhibit targets which are very valuable in the optimization of lead compounds (Morris and Lim-Wilby 2008).

Molecular docking simulation is divided into three main protocols, namely induced-fit, lock and key, and ensemble docking. Induced-fit docking occurs when a ligand flexibly binds to the active sites of protein in order to maximize bonding strength, usually called flexible docking. While the lock and key, often referred to as rigid docking, is the type of simulation where the protein in a rigid condition and ligand move continuously to find its optimal conformation. Lastly, there is ensemble docking which can explain the flexibility and complexity of the state of protein conformation (Tripathi and Misra 2017). Rigid and flexible docking simulation using Molecular Operating Environment (MOE) software is the most common method used for drug design from our lab. Energy interactions between ligands and protein targets are calculated using electrostatic and van der Waals potential fields (Vilar, Cozza, and Moro 2008).

The following are examples of the successful CADD application passed through the clinical trial stage or approved for therapeutic use such as captopril, zanamivir, boceprevir, oseltamivir, rupintrivir, saquinavir, dorzolamide, aliskiren, nolatrexed, MI-005, LY-517717, and NVP-AUY922 (Talele, Khedkar, and Rigby 2010). The computational study for developing Ebola drug was conducted by Setlur et al. through the screening process of ligands from natural compounds and predicting the binding potential for VP24, VP30, VP35, and VP40 protein targets. In the preparation stage, the crystal structures from each protein were retrieved from the PDB database, then verified using the Ramachandran Plot. Moreover, all water molecules and associated heteroatoms were removed from the original protein structures, then polar hydrogen atoms were added together with the Kollman charges. In the ligand preparation process, all compounds from Indian medicinal plants must be screened to eliminate the compounds which did not qualify the druglikeness and ADMET properties. Only the prepared and optimized ligands were used for molecular docking simulation (Setlur, Naik, and Skariyachan 2017).

About 35 selected natural ligands underwent the molecular docking simulation for each receptor by utilizing AutoDock Vina. Limonin is the best ligand for VP24 and VP35 protein, with the binding energy of -9.70 kcal/mol. Meanwhile, curcumin and mahanine exhibited the minimum theoretical binding energy of -9.60 and -7.70 kcal/mol, respectively. The ligands play an essential role to inhibit the activity of several Virion Protein (VP) of Ebola virus. In addition, the presence of hydrogen bonds interaction between protein and the phytoligand makes the ligand binding position more stable. Although wet laboratory experiments are urgently needed, current data will certainly open the way for drug discovery various deadly viral diseases (Setlur, Naik, and Skariyachan 2017).

Natural product compounds still a preferable choice for ligand candidate. The flavonoid (gossypetin and taxifolin) as one of the classes of natural product compounds through virtual screening and molecular docking studies have shown better docking scores and energy binding value in all the EBOV receptor (VP40, VP35, VP30, and VP24) (Raj and Varadwaj 2016). Besides flavonoids, natural compounds contained in

Traditional Chinese Medicine (TCM) is also often used in the fields of medical diagnosis and treatment. The TCM database composes more than 20,000 pure compounds isolated from 453 TCM ingredients which are suitable to download for virtual screening in 2D or 3D formats (Chen 2011). The research using the TCM database found that emodin-8-beta-D-glucoside could inhibit the activity of VP40 through interaction with the key residues for RNA binding. Moreover, emodin-8-O-beta-D-glucoside which is extracted from the herb *Polygonum cuspidatum* shows excellent pharmacokinetic properties based on ADME and drug-likeness analysis (Karthick et al. 2016).

Computational-based EVD drug discovery was also conducted through the repurposing of some medicinal for inhibiting Ebola virus protein. The signaling pathway activation of TGF-β1 by Ebola virus has a vital role in the EVD pathogenesis. Ibuprofen as a drug with minimal toxic was repurposed as an inhibitor of the Ebola GP1. As an inhibitor, ibuprofen could prevent GP1/EMILIN-1 interaction allowing EMILIN-1 for keeping control of the TGF-β1 signaling pathway (Veljkovic et al. 2015). Further investigation of ibuprofen as inhibitor EBOV protein must be evaluated, so the drug becomes a promising drug which is low- toxic, inexpensive and wide-accessible candidates for the treatment of EVD.

ABOUT OUR RESEARCH

The objective of this chapter is to review the successful developed drug candidates to treat EVD by using EBOV protein structure, such as VP24, VP35, VP40, nucleoprotein, and glycoprotein. The research studies followed the pipeline procedure that was developed from our research group. Proteins and ligands must be prepared and optimized by using MOE 2014.09 software before performing molecular docking simulation. The best ligands must fulfill the requirements such as attaching to the binding sites of protein, have Gibbs Free Binding Energy (ΔG binding) score lower than standard ligand, and shown preferable interaction with the protein. Furthermore, some drug candidates from in silico study also undergo pharmacokinetic analysis by using any software to suppress possible failure when evaluated in the wet laboratory.

VP24

EBOV VP24 is a secondary matrix protein which localizes in the plasma membrane and perinuclear region in both transfected and EBOV-infected cells. VP24 has an important role during virus assembly and budding which make the protein become a potential target to combat EVD (Han et al. 2003). In this study, Indonesian natural product compounds from HerbalDB database were used to inhibit VP24 protein (Yanuar et al. 2014). About 2,020 compounds redrawn before being filtered to fulfil Lipinski's rule of five (RO5), Veber's rule, and druglikeness score as well as filtering potentially toxic compounds by using DataWarrior software.

Lipinski and Veber regulate the physicochemical characteristics of drugs in order to produce proper absorption, permeation and bioavailability, if following criteria such as molecular weight less than 500Da, logP less than 5, hydrogen bond donor less than 5, hydrogen bond acceptor less than 10, rotatable bonds less than 10, and polar surface area equal to or less than 140 Å^2. However, this rule does not apply to biological transporter or natural substrates (Bickerton et al. 2012; Veber et al. 2002). While Quantitative Estimate of Druglikeness (QED) that have developed by Hopkins sets druglikeness score more than zero as the main consideration for selecting compounds at the early stage drug discovery which related to solubility, permeability, metabolic stability, and transporter effects of molecular behavior in vivo (Bickerton et al. 2012).

Inhibitor of EBOV VP24 was produced through the molecular docking simulation between protein structure (PDB ID: 4M0Q) and the ligands. The best ligand is cycloartocarpin which attaches to the binding sites of EBOV VP24 protein (Gln103, Leu106, Gly117, Gly120, Leu121, Ser123, Asp124, Leu127, Thr128, Thr183, Gln184, Asn185, and His186) and has the ΔG binding value lower than the standard (- 7.48 kcal/mol) (U.S.F.

Tambunan and Nasution 2017). This ligand forms a hydrogen bond interaction with Gln109 residue, as shown as in Figure 1.

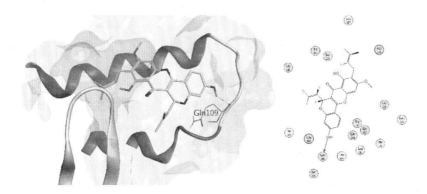

Figure 1. Molecular interaction of cycloartocarpin with EBOV VP24 protein.

Beside using Indonesian natural product compounds as the inhibitor of EBOV VP24 protein, the study also applied an in vitro drug-series of ZINC15 database (Sterling and Irwin 2015). The other study used FBDD as the main approach. All compounds obtained from the database must be filtered according to the Rules of Three and toxicity screening assay by using DataWarrior software. Fragment linking method was utilized to generate potential ligands that can inhibit VP24 protein (PDB ID: 4U2X) (U.S.F. Tambunan, Siregar, and Toepak 2018).

About 1,285 selected fragments underwent rigid docking simulation to obtain ΔG binding score which is used to predict the conformation of the ligand-protein that binds stronger. Fragments 1266 and 440 were chosen to conduct fragment linking using 'Link Multiple Fragments' feature in MOE software. Furthermore, the redocking process include rigid and flexible docking was carried out between the linker fragment and protein. Rigid docking was conducted for eliminating the low affinity and bad pose of ligands while flexible docking was performed to observe the molecular interaction and binding affinity from selected ligands (Putra et al. 2018).

The best ligand (L595) has ΔG binding value of - 54.26 kcal/mol that was obtained from the redocking process through molecular interaction with Leu201, Lys218, Leu127, Ser89, Trp38, Leu91, Trp92, Thr128,

Thr129, Asn130, Glu88, Val31, Asn132, and Leu91 residues. In Figure 2, there is more molecular interaction between VP24 protein and L595 compared with cycloartocarpin. L595 has a lower ΔG binding value due to this ligand is established through fragment linking where the fragments were linked directly to the active sites of the protein.

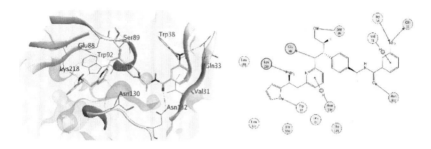

Figure 2. Molecular interaction of L595 with EBOV VP24 protein.

The toxicity prediction of L595 indicated that this molecule does not give reproductive effect, mutagenic and carcinogenic potency based on VEGA and Toxtree analysis. Also, according to molecular dynamics simulation at 312K for 20,000 ps (picosecond), L595 has more stable interaction compared to all ligands and standard. Thus, L595 become a promising drug candidate for against EBOV (U.S.F. Tambunan, Siregar, and Toepak 2018).

VP35

As a multifunctional protein, VP35 serves as an essential cofactor of the viral RNA polymerase complex, an innate immune antagonist, an RNAi silencing suppressor, and an enzyme required for viral assembly (Leung et al. 2010). VP35 is a potential target for against EBOV because the protein was detected as an interferon antagonist that may contribute to the virulence of EBOV (Basler et al. 2000). The protein structure with PDB ID: 3FKE was used as receptor atom while biogenic compounds from

ZINC15 database were applied as the ligand candidate (Sterling and Irwin 2015; Imani et al. 1988).

The research used fragment linking method for drug discovery, as the previous discussion. Around 6,662 fragments were filtered from the biogenic compound of ZINC15 database based on the Astex Rules of Three and toxicity filter. Furthermore, two potential fragments from docking simulation that do not overlap and have Root Mean Square Deviation (RMSD) less than 2Å were selected for the linker process using MOE software. After the redocking simulation, three of 91 ligands as linker result have been selected as a drug candidate for EVD. However, among all ligand, LEB 31 was chosen as the best ligand due to the lowest ΔG binding value of -50.54 kcal/mol (Marnolia, Toepak, and Tambunan 2018). Some amino acid residues that interact in complex protein-ligand are Gln241, Gln244, Lys248, Lys251, Arg225, Ala221, Tyr229, Lys222, Phe235, Pro304 (Figure 3). Six main residues establish important molecular interactions, including Phe235, Lys251, Ala221, Arg225, Gln244, and Gln241.

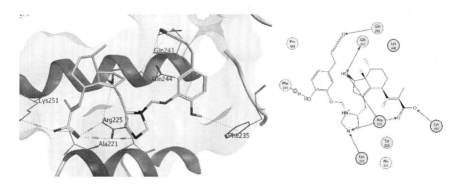

Figure 3. Molecular interaction of LEB 31 with EBOV VP35 protein.

In addition to having the lowest ΔG binding value among all ligands and standard, LEB 31 also contains no reproductive toxicity, mutagen, and carcinogen properties. Moreover, molecular dynamics simulation shows that LEB 31 is the most stable an average RMSD of 0.50 Å (Marnolia, Toepak, and Tambunan 2018).

The application of the VP35 protein in the drug design against EBOV was discussed in the previous book chapter (Usman Sumo Friend Tambunan, Alkaff, and Nasution 2018). Protein structure with PDB ID: 4IBC used as a receptor and Indonesian natural product compounds as the ligand candidates. The study used pharmacophore based molecular docking, wherein the process docking performed by applying pharmacophore features which have been obtained through the standard Protein-Ligand Interaction Fingerprints (PLIF) protocol in MOE software. Pharmacophores are used to determine important features of one or more molecules, usually from the standard drug, with the same biological activity. The characteristic of the pharmacophore feature is where molecules have hydrophobic, aromatic, hydrogen bond acceptor, hydrogen bonding, cation or anion interaction with the receptor (Gao, Yang, and Zhu 2010).

From 3,429 initial compounds, only 20 ligands that matched with the pharmacophore features of the protein. After molecular docking simulation, the best ligands with the lowest ΔG binding score is multifloroside with a score of - 10.84 kcal/mol. However, the RMSD value of multifloroside molecule is higher than 2.0 Å (3.26 Å) which means the docking pose generated during the docking simulation was unacceptable. Hence, the second lowest ligand, myricetin 3-robinobioside was selected as a drug candidate for EVD due to the preferable RMSD value of 1.22 Å (Tambunan, Alkaff, and Nasution 2018).

VP40

Matrix protein VP40 of EBOV is widely expressed during filoviral infection and plays some important roles in the life cycle of filoviruses, such as regulating the transcription of viral protein and coordinating virion assembly and budding from infected cells. As a result, inhibition of EBOV VP40 become an extremely promising therapeutic strategy for control EVD (Madara et al. 2015).

Indonesian natural product compound were applied for obtaining VP40 inhibitor (M. A.F. Nasution, Alkaff, and Tambunan 2018). On the other side, protein structure with PDB ID: 4LDB was used as a template represented EBOV VP40 protein (Bornholdt et al. 2013). As standard procedure for ligand preparation using DataWarrior, about 3,429 Indonesian natural product compounds that collected from several sources underwent screening based on toxicity properties and druglikeness score. Only 527 ligands were used later in the molecular docking simulation.

Using MOE software, docking simulation was performed to predict the conformation of a ligand when to fit into the binding site of the protein selected by employing 'Site Finder' feature. Mesuaferrone B as the best ligand having the lowest ΔG binding value of -8.60 kcal/mol and RMSD of 1.11 Å. According to molecular interaction, the ligand has three hydrogen bond interactions with Leu98, Asp193, and Pro286 residues along with three aromatic pi-pi (π-π) interactions on Arg151, Ile216, and Leu217 residues (M. A. F. Nasution, Alkaff, and Tambunan 2018). All molecular interaction is shown in Figure 4.

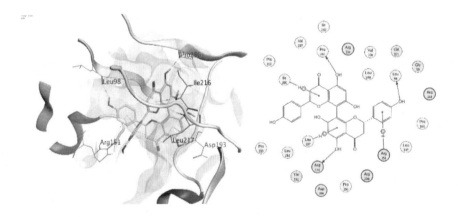

Figure 4. Molecular interaction of mesuaferrone B with EBOV VP40 protein.

Nucleoprotein

Beside using virion protein, nucleoprotein also becomes a potential target in drug development against EBOV. The EBOV nucleoprotein (NP) is the largest among the nonsegmented negative-stranded RNA viruses which separated into a hydrophobic N-terminal half and a hydrophilic C-terminal half (Watanabe, Noda, and Kawaoka 2006). Role of the NP is to facilitate the encapsidation genomic RNA to form viral ribonucleoprotein (RNP) complex together with genome RNA and polymerase. This complex has the most crucial role in virus proliferation cycle so the inhibition its work become an attractive target for the antiviral development of EBOV (Dong et al. 2015).

The research study was still based on the computational approach, where the protein structure was obtained from RCSB PDB with PDB ID: 4Z9P and natural product compounds from ZINC15 database were used as the ligands candidate (Dong et al. 2015; Sterling and Irwin 2015). Prior to uses, the compounds were filtered based on Lipinski's Rule of Five (RO5) and Veber's rule (with several exceptions), toxicity potency, and druglikeness score. Using MOE software, about 3,884 of 190,084 compounds underwent the optimization and energy minimization steps along with the protein structure so that it can be continued to molecular docking simulation.

From the docking simulation, ten ligands were selected due to their lower ΔG binding value compared to standard. However, ZINC85628951 is the best drug candidate for targeting EBOV NP which has ΔG binding value of - 7.28 kcal/mol and RMSD of 1.79 Å. Molecular interaction between ZINC85628951 and EBOV NP was also observed by using 'Ligand Interaction' feature on MOE software. As shown in Figure 5, this ligand has some interactions such as pi-pi, hydrogen bond, and van der Waals interaction. The most crucial interactions to become the inhibitor of EBOV NP are interactions on Arg298 and His310 residues which are two of the RNA binding groove site residues.

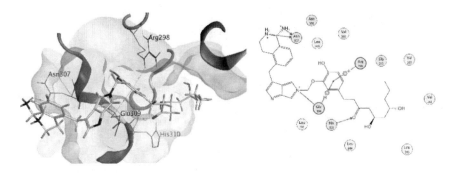

Figure 5. Molecular interaction of ZINC85628951 with EBOV NP.

The pharmacokinetics analysis reveals that ZINC85628951 well absorbed in gastrointestinal and has bioavailability score of 0.55 which was considered as good. Moreover, the ligand does not inhibit the work of cytochrome P450 that act as enzyme for drug metabolism. The toxicity prediction shows that the ligand does not contain both genotoxic and non-genotoxic carcinogenicity. In addition, the potential Salmonella typhimurium TA100 mutagen and potential carcinogen based on QSAR are also not detected in the ligand (Mochammad Arfin Fardiansyah Nasution et al. 2018).

Glycoprotein

EBOV enter the host through mucosal surfaces, abrasions, and injuries in the skin or by parental transmission (Feldmann and Geisbert 2011). EBOV binds to a receptor on the cell surface for then internalized through macropinocytosis and trafficked to endosomal compartments by using glycoprotein. In endosome, glycoprotein was digested cysteine proteases cathepsin B (CatB) and cathepsin L (CatL) to form a 19 kDa viral glycoprotein (GP2). The fusion between the viral and endosomal membranes resulted when GP2 interacts with Niemann-Pick C1 (NPC1). Furthermore, the viral nucleocapsid is delivered into the cytoplasm for replication (Falasca et al. 2015). Therefore, molecules which can inhibit GP activity become an ideal medicinal treatment for Ebola virus disease.

Besides *Zaire ebolavirus*, *Sudan ebolavirus* (SEBOV) becomes the second deadliest *ebolavirus* with the fatality rate of 50 - 70%. The study conducted by Putra et al., utilizing the crystal structure of SEBOV GP with PDB ID: 3VE0 as the receptor. Using NCBI BLAST, SEBOV glycoprotein is detected 99.6% of similarity from the other *ebolavirus*. Flavonoid compounds from the ChEBI database as selected as the source of candidate ligands. Flavonoid which is easily found in various plants, fruits, and vegetables be trusted has low toxicity, high on the bioavailability and antioxidant activity, as well as free radical activity. For finding the best ligand as the drug candidate that can inhibit the activity of SEBOV GP, both molecular docking simulation and computational ADMET test was applied (Putra et al. 2018).

From 1,358 selected compounds from the previous analysis, only 7 flavonoid compounds that chosen to become the best ligand according to molecular docking result considering the ability to be attached to the binding site of GP protein and have a higher binding affinity proven by having lower ΔG binding value than the standard ligands. Among all best ligands, cyanidin-3-(p-coumaroyl)-rutinoside-5-glucoside has the lowest ΔG binding value of - 9.69 kcal/mol. However, the RMSD score of this molecule (3.17 Å) shows that the pose that formed during the docking simulation is unacceptable. Therefore, myrciatrin V is preferred to become an EVD drug candidate that has ΔG binding value of - 9.17 kcal/mol and RMSD score of 1.83 Å.

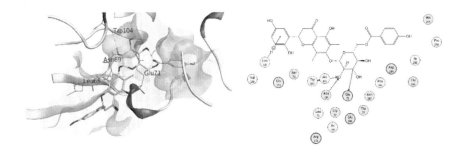

Figure 6. Molecular interaction of myrciacitrin V with SEBOV GP.

As shown in Figure 6, myrciacitrin V establish hydrogen bond interactions at Trp104, Glu71 and Gly72 residues and hydrogen-arene interaction with Leu68 residue. Furthermore, the ligand was also predicted as safe drug candidates seen from the absence of mutagenic, tumorigenic, effective reproductive, and irritant potential (Putra et al. 2018).

CONCLUSION

Considering the high mortality rate due to EBOV infection makes the drugs discovery and development become an urgent necessity that must be done. In this chapter, we have reviewed the ability of bioinformatics study through the CADD to design drug candidates at an early stage and predicting the feasibility of these lead compounds. Feasibility prediction of the drug is important due to many lead compounds failed to be continued in the next stage due to poor pharmacokinetics, safety, and efficacy. The toxicity prediction such as mutagenic, carcinogen, tumorigenic, irritants, and reproductive effects are the most essential for human.

Natural product compounds are still the most preferred choice for drug candidate due to the easier to find in nature and have fewer side effects. From the overall research studies that have done in our lab, it can be seen that the FBDD method can produce inhibitors that have the lowest energy binding. However, the difficulty of synthesis process still becomes the main consideration if compared to the purification process of natural product compounds. Further research such as *in vitro*, *in vivo* and clinical study must be conducted to evaluate the results previously obtained.

REFERENCES

Allela, Loïs., Olivier, Boury., Régis, Pouillot., André, Délicat., Philippe, Yaba., Brice, Kumulungui., Pierre, Rouquet., Jean-Paul, Gonzalez. & Eric, M. Leroy. (2005). "Ebola Virus Antibody Prevalence in Dogs and Human Risk." *Emerging Infectious Diseases*, *11* (3), 385–90. https:// doi.org/10.3201/eid1103.040981.

Basler, Christopher F., Xiuyan, Wang., Elke, Mü Hlberger†., Victor, Volchkov., Jason, Paragas., Hans-Dieter, Klenk., Adolfo, García-Sastre. & Peter, Palese. (2000). "The Ebola Virus VP35 Protein Functions as a Type I IFN Antagonist." *Proceedings of the National Academy of Sciences of the United States of America*, *97* (22), 12289–94. https://doi.org/10.1073/pnas.220398297.

Bausch, Daniel G., Jonathan, S. Towner., Scott, F. Dowell., Felix, Kaducu., Matthew, Lukwiya., Anthony, Sanchez., Stuart, T. Nichol., Thomas, G. Ksiazek. & Pierre, E. Rollin. (2007). "Assessment of the Risk of Ebola Virus Transmission from Bodily Fluids and Fomites." *The Journal of Infectious Diseases*, *196* (Suppl2), S142–47. https:// doi.org/10.1086/520545.

Bell, Beth P., Inger, K. Damon., Daniel, B. Jernigan., Thomas, A. Kenyon., Stuart, T. Nichol., John, P. O'Connor. & Jordan, W. Tappero. (2016). "Overview, Control Strategies, and Lessons Learned in the CDC Response to the 2014–2016 Ebola Epidemic." *MMWR Supplements*, *65* (3), 4–11. https://doi.org/10.15585/mmwr.su6503a2.

Bickerton, G Richard., Gaia, V. Paolini., Jérémy, Besnard., Sorel, Muresan. & Andrew, L Hopkins. (2012). "Quantifying the Chemical Beauty of Drugs." *Nature Chemistry*, *4* (2), 90–98. https://doi.org/10.1038/ nchem.1243.

Bixler, Sandra L., Thomas, M. Bocan., Jay, Wells., Kelly, S. Wetzel., Sean, A. Van Tongeren., Lian, Dong., Nicole, L. Garza., et al. (2018). "Efficacy of Favipiravir (T-705) in Nonhuman Primates Infected with Ebola Virus or Marburg Virus." *Antiviral Research*, *151*, 97–104. https://doi.org/10.1016/j.antiviral.2017.12.021.

Bixler, Sandra L., Allen, J. Duplantier. & Sina, Bavari. (2017). "Discovering Drugs for the Treatment of Ebola Virus." *Current Treatment Options in Infectious Diseases*, *9* (3), 299–317. https://doi. org/10.1007/s40506-017-0130-z.

Bornholdt, Zachary A., Takeshi, Noda., Dafna, M. Abelson., Peter, Halfmann., Malcolm, R. Wood., Yoshihiro, Kawaoka. & Erica,

Ollmann Saphire. (2013). "Structural Rearrangement of Ebola Virus VP40 Begets Multiple Functions in the Virus Life Cycle." *Cell, 154* (4), 763–74. https://doi.org/10.1016/j.cell.2013.07.015.

Centers for Disease Control and Prevention. (2018). "Ebola (Ebola Virus Disease)." 2018. https://www.cdc.gov/vhf/ebola/about.html.

Chen, Calvin Yu-Chian. (2011). "TCM Database@Taiwan: The World's Largest Traditional Chinese Medicine Database for Drug Screening in Silico." *PloS One, 6* (1), e15939. https://doi.org/10.1371/journal. pone.0015939.

Congreve, Miles., Robin, Carr., Chris, Murray. & Harren, Jhoti. (2003). "A 'Rule of Three' for Fragment-Based Lead Discovery?" *Drug Discovery Today, 8* (19), 876–77. https://doi.org/10.1016/S1359-6446(03)02831-9.

Davey, Richard T., Lori, Dodd., Michael, A. Proschan., James, Neaton., Jacquie, Neuhaus Nordwall., Joseph, S. Koopmeiners., John, Beigel., et al. (2016). "A Randomized, Controlled Trial of ZMapp for Ebola Virus Infection." *New England Journal of Medicine, 375* (15), 1448–56. https://doi.org/10.1056/NEJMoa1604330.

Dong, Shishang., Peng, Yang., Guobang, Li., Baocheng, Liu., Wenming, Wang., Xiang, Liu., Boran, Xia., et al. (2015). "Insight into the Ebola Virus Nucleocapsid Assembly Mechanism: Crystal Structure of Ebola Virus Nucleoprotein Core Domain at 1.8 Å Resolution." *Protein & Cell, 6* (5), 351–62. https://doi.org/10.1007/s13238-015-0163-3.

Dowall, Stuart D., Andrew, Bosworth., Robert, Watson., Kevin, Bewley., Irene, Taylor., Emma, Rayner., Laura, Hunter., et al. (2015). "Chloroquine Inhibited Ebola Virus Replication *in Vitro* but Failed to Protect against Infection and Disease in the *in Vivo* Guinea Pig Model." *Journal of General Virology, 96* (12), 3484–92. https://doi.org/10.1099/jgv.0.000309.

Dunning, Jake., Foday, Sahr., Amanda, Rojek., Fiona, Gannon., Gail, Carson, Baimba Idriss., Thomas, Massaquoi., et al. (2016). "Experimental Treatment of Ebola Virus Disease with TKM-130803: A Single-Arm Phase 2 Clinical Trial." Edited by Lorenz von Seidlein.

PLOS Medicine, *13* (4), e1001997. https://doi.org/10.1371/journal.pmed.1001997.

Erlanson, Daniel A., Robert, S. McDowell. & Tom, O'Brien. (2004). "Fragment-Based Drug Discovery." *Journal of Medicinal Chemistry*, *47* (14), 3463–82. https://doi.org/10.1021/jm040031v.

Falasca, L., Agrati, C., Petrosillo, N., Di Caro, A., Capobianchi, M. R., Ippolito, G. & Piacentini, M. (2015). "Molecular Mechanisms of Ebola Virus Pathogenesis: Focus on Cell Death." *Cell Death and Differentiation*, *22*, 1250–59. https://doi.org/10.1038/cdd.2015.67.

Feldmann, Heinz. & Thomas, W. Geisbert. (2011). "Ebola Haemorrhagic Fever." *Lancet*, *377* (9768), 849–62. https://doi.org/10.1016/S0140-6736(10)60667-8.

Ferreira, Leonardo G., Ricardo, N. Dos Santos., Glaucius, Oliva. & Adriano, D. Andricopulo. (2015). "Molecular Docking and Structure-Based Drug Design Strategies." *Molecules*, *20* (7), 13384–421. https://doi.org/10.3390/molecules200713384.

Gao, Qingzhi., Lulu, Yang. & Yongqiang, Zhu. (2010). "Pharmacophore Based Drug Design Approach as a Practical Process in Drug Discovery." *Current Computer Aided-Drug Design*, *6* (1), 37–49. https://doi.org/10.2174/157340910790980151.

García-Dorival, Isabel., Weining, Wu., Stuart, Dowall., Stuart, Armstrong., Olivier, Touzelet., Jonathan, Wastling., John, N. Barr., et al. (2014). "Elucidation of the Ebola Virus VP24 Cellular Interactome and Disruption of Virus Biology through Targeted Inhibition of Host-Cell Protein Function." *Journal of Proteome Research*, *13*, 5120–35. https://doi.org/10.1021/pr500556d.

Geisbert, Thomas W., Lisa, E. Hensley., Elliott, Kagan., Erik, Zhaoying Yu., Joan, B. Geisbert., Kathleen, Daddario-DiCaprio., Elizabeth, A. Fritz., et al. (2006). "Postexposure Protection of Guinea Pigs against a Lethal Ebola Virus Challenge Is Conferred by RNA Interference." *The Journal of Infectious Diseases*, *193* (12), 1650–57. https://doi.org/10.1086/504267.

Geisbert, Thomas W., Amy, C. H. Lee., Marjorie, Robbins., Joan, B Geisbert., Anna, N. Honko., Vandana, Sood., Joshua, C. Johnson., et al. (2010). "Postexposure Protection of Non-Human Primates against a Lethal Ebola Virus Challenge with RNA Interference: A Proof-of-Concept Study." *The Lancet*, *375* (9729), 1896–1905. https://doi.org/ 10.1016/S0140-6736(10)60357-1.

Han, Ziying., Hani, Boshra., Oriol Sunyer, J., Susan, H Zwiers., Jason, Paragas. & Ronald, N Harty. (2003). "Biochemical and Functional Characterization of the Ebola Virus VP24 Protein: Implications for a Role in Virus Assembly and Budding." *Journal of Virology*, *77* (3), 1793–1800. https://doi.org/10.1128/JVI.77.3.1793-1800.2003.

Hoenen, Thomas., Allison, Groseth., Darryl, Falzarano. & Heinz, Feldmann. (2006). "Ebola Virus: Unravelling Pathogenesis to Combat a Deadly Disease." *Trends in Molecular Medicine*, *12* (5), 206–15. https://doi.org/10.1016/j.molmed.2006.03.006.

Huang, Hung Jin., Hsin, Wei Yu., Chien, Yu Chen., Chih, Ho Hsu., Hsin, Yi Chen., Kuei, Jen Lee., Fuu, Jen Tsai. & Calvin, Yu Chian Chen. (2010). "Current Developments of Computer-Aided Drug Design." *Journal of the Taiwan Institute of Chemical Engineers*, *41* (6), 623–35. https://doi.org/10.1016/j.jtice.2010.03.017.

Imani, F., Jacobs, B. L., Bruce Fulton, D., Jay, Nix., Christopher, F. Basler., Richard, B. Honzatko. & Gaya, K. Amarasinghe. (1988). "Inhibitory Activity for the Interferon-Induced Protein Kinase Is Associated with the Reovirus Serotype 1 Sigma 3 Protein." *Proceedings of the National Academy of Sciences of the United States of America*, *85* (21), 7887–91. https://doi.org/10.1073/pnas.85. 21.7887.

Iversen, Patrick L., Travis, K. Warren., Jay, B. Wells., Nicole, L. Garza., Dan, V. Mourich., Lisa, S. Welch., Rekha, G. Panchal. & Sina, Bavari. (2012). "Discovery and Early Development of AVI-7537 and AVI-7288 for the Treatment of Ebola Virus and Marburg Virus Infections." *Viruses*, *4*, 2806–30. https://doi.org/10.3390/v4112806.

Judson, Seth., Joseph, Prescott. & Vincent, Munster. (2015). "Understanding Ebola Virus Transmission." *Viruses*, *7* (2), 511–21. https://doi.org/10.3390/v7020511.

Karthick, V., Nagasundaram, N., George Priya Doss, C., Chiranjib, Chakraborty., Siva, R., Aiping, Lu., Ge, Zhang. & Hailong, Zhu. (2016). "Virtual Screening of the Inhibitors Targeting at the Viral Protein 40 of Ebola Virus." *Infectious Diseases of Poverty*, *5* (1), 12. https://doi.org/10.1186/s40249-016-0105-1.

Leligdowicz, Aleksandra., William, A. Fischer., Timothy, M. Uyeki., Thomas, E. Fletcher., Neill, K. J. Adhikari., Gina, Portella., Francois, Lamontagne., et al. (2016). "Ebola Virus Disease and Critical Illness." *Critical Care*, *20* (1), 217. https://doi.org/10.1186/s13054-016-1325-2.

Leroy, Eric M., Brice, Kumulungui., Xavier, Pourrut., Pierre, Rouquet., Alexandre, Hassanin., Philippe, Yaba., André, Délicat., Janusz, T. Paweska., Jean-Paul, Gonzalez. & Robert, Swanepoel. (2005). "Fruit Bats as Reservoirs of Ebola Virus." *Nature*, *438* (7068), 575–76. https://doi.org/10.1038/438575a.

Leung, Daisy W., Kathleen, C. Prins., Christopher, F. Basler. & Gaya, K. Amarasinghe. (2010). "Ebolavirus VP35 Is a Multifunctional Virulence Factor." *Virulence*, *1* (6), 526–31. https://doi.org/10.4161/ VIRU.1.6.12984.

MacNeil, Adam. & Pierre, E. Rollin. (2012). "Ebola and Marburg Hemorrhagic Fevers: Neglected Tropical Diseases?" Edited by Thomas Geisbert. *PLoS Neglected Tropical Diseases*, *6* (6), e1546. https://doi.org/10.1371/journal.pntd.0001546.

Madara, Jonathan J., Ziying, Han., Gordon, Ruthel., Bruce, D. Freedman. & Ronald, N. Harty. (2015). "The Multifunctional Ebola Virus VP40 Matrix Protein Is a Promising Therapeutic Target." *Future Virol*, *10* (5), 537–46. https://doi.org/10.2217/fvl.15.6.

Malvy, Denis., Anita, K McElroy., Hilde, de Clerck., Stephan, Günther. & Johan, van Griensven. (2019). "Ebola Virus Disease." *Lancet*, *393* (10174), 936–48. https://doi.org/10.1016/S0140-6736(18)33132-5.

Marnolia, Atika., Erwin, Prasetya Toepak. & Usman, Sumo Friend Tambunan. (2018). "Fragment-Based Lead Compound Design To Inhibit Ebola VP35 Through Computational Studies." *International Journal of GEOMATE*, *15* (49), 65–71. https://doi.org/10.21660/ 2018.49.3535.

Mehedi, Masfique., Darryl, Falzarano., Jochen, Seebach., Xiaojie, Hu., Michael, S. Carpenter., Hans-Joachim, Schnittler. & Heinz, Feldmann. (2011). "A New Ebola Virus Nonstructural Glycoprotein Expressed through RNA Editing." *Journal of Virology*, *85* (11), 5406–14. https://doi.org/10.1128/JVI.02190-10.

Meng, Xuan-Yu., Hong-Xing, Zhang., Mihaly, Mezei. & Meng, Cui. (2011). "Molecular Docking: A Powerful Approach for Structure-Based Drug Discovery." *Current Computer Aided Drug Design*, *7* (2), 146–157. https://www.ncbi.nlm.nih.gov/pmc/articles/ PMC3151162/pdf/nihms-308746.pdf.

Morris, Garrett M. & Marguerita, Lim-Wilby. (2008). "Molecular Docking." In *Methods in Molecular Biology*, *443*, 365–82. Springer. https://doi.org/10.1007/978-1-59745-177-2_19.

Nasution, M. A. F., Alkaff, A. H. & Tambunan, U. S. F. (2018). "Discovery of Indonesian Natural Products as Potential Inhibitor of Ebola Virus VP40 through Molecular Docking Simulation." *AIP Conference Proceedings*, *2023* (20055), 1–6. https://doi.org/10.1063/1.5064052.

Nasution, Mochammad Arfin Fardiansyah., Erwin, Prasetya Toepak., Ahmad, Husein Alkaff. & Usman, Sumo Friend Tambunan. (2018). "Flexible Docking-Based Molecular Dynamics Simulation of Natural Product Compounds and Ebola Virus Nucleocapsid (EBOV NP): A Computational Approach to Discover New Drug for Combating Ebola." *BMC Bioinformatics*, *19* (419), 137–49. https://doi.org/10.1186/s12859-018-2387-8.

Patterson, Marc C., Darleen, Vecchio., Helena, Prady., Larry, Abel. & James, E. Wraith. (2007). "Miglustat for Treatment of Niemann-Pick C Disease: A Randomised Controlled Study." *The Lancet Neurology*, *6* (9), 765–72. https://doi.org/10.1016/S1474-4422(07)70194-1.

Putra, Rendy Pramuda., Ahmad, Husein Alkaff., Fardiansyah Nasution, M. A., Agustinus, C. B. Kantale. & Tambunan, U. S. F. (2018). "Searching of Flavonoid Compounds as a New Antiviral for Sudan Ebolavirus Glycoprotein Using in Silico Methods." *International*

Journal of GEOMATE, Sept, 15 (49), 78–84. https://doi.org/10.21660/ 2018.49. 3606.

Raj, Utkarsh. & Pritish, Kumar Varadwaj. (2016). "Flavonoids as Multi-Target Inhibitors for Proteins Associated with Ebola Virus: In Silico Discovery Using Virtual Screening and Molecular Docking Studies." *Interdisciplinary Sciences: Computational Life Sciences, 8* (2), 132–41. https://doi.org/10.1007/s12539-015-0109-8.

Salazar, Daniel E. & Glenn, Gormley. (2017). "Modern Drug Discovery and Development." In *Clinical and Translational Science*, 719–43. Elsevier. https://doi.org/10.1016/B978-0-12-802101-9.00041-7.

Scott, Duncan E., Anthony, G. Coyne., Sean, A. Hudson. & Chris, Abell. (2012). "Fragment-Based Approaches in Drug Discovery and Chemical Biology." *Biochemistry, 51* (25), 4990–5003. https://doi.org/10.4137/ DTI.S31566.

Setlur, Anagha S., Sujay, Y. Naik. & Sinosh, Skariyachan. (2017). "Herbal Lead as Ideal Bioactive Compounds Against Probable Drug Targets of Ebola Virus in Comparison with Known Chemical Analogue: A Computational Drug Discovery Perspective." *Interdisciplinary Sciences: Computational Life Sciences, 9* (2), 254–77. https://doi.org/ 10.1007/s12539-016-0149-8.

Sterling, Teague. & John, J. Irwin. (2015). "ZINC 15-Ligand Discovery for Everyone." *Journal of Chemical Information and Modeling, 55* (11), 2324–37. https://doi.org/10.1021/acs.jcim.5b00559.

Talele, Tanaji., Santosh, Khedkar. & Alan, Rigby. (2010). "Successful Applications of Computer Aided Drug Discovery: Moving Drugs from Concept to the Clinic." *Current Topics in Medicinal Chemistry, 10* (1), 127–41. https://doi.org/10.2174/156802610790232251.

Tambunan, U. S. F. & Nasution, M. A. F. (2017). "Identification of Novel Ebola Virus (EBOV) VP24 Inhibitor from Indonesian Natural Products through in Silico Drug Design Approach." *AIP Conference Proceedings, 1862* (30091), 1–9. https://doi.org/10.1063/1.4991195.

Tambunan, U. S. F., Syafrida, Siregar. & Erwin, Prasetya Toepak. (2018). "Ebola Viral Protein 24 (VP24) Inhibitor Discovery by In Silico

Fragment-Based Design." *International Journal of GEOMATE*, *15* (49), 59–64. https://doi.org/10.21660/2018.49.3534.

Tambunan, Usman Sumo Friend., Ahmad, Husein Alkaff. & Mochammad, Arfin Fardiansyah Nasution. (2018). "Bioinformatics Approach to Screening and Developing Drug against Ebola." In *Advances in Ebola Control*, 75–88. IntechOpen. https://doi.org/10.5772/intechopen.72278 Abstract.

Taylor, Raymond., Pravin, Kotian., Travis, Warren., Rekha, Panchal., Sina, Bavari., Justin, Julander., Sylvia, Dobo., et al. (2016). "BCX4430 – A Broad-Spectrum Antiviral Adenosine Nucleoside Analog under Development for the Treatment of Ebola Virus Disease." *Journal of Infection and Public Health*, *9* (3), 220–26. https://doi.org/10.1016/j.jiph.2016.04.002.

Teufel, Andreas., Markus, Krupp., Arndt, Weinmann. & Peter, R. Galle. (2006). "Current Bioinformatics Tools in Genomic Biomedical Research (Review)." *International Journal of Molecular Medicine*, *17* (6), 967–73.

Torre, Giuseppe La., Vincenzo, Nicosia. & Maurizio, Cardi. (2014). "Ebola: A Review on the State of the Art on Prevention and Treatment." *Asian Pacific Journal of Tropical Biomedicine*, *4* (12), 925–27. https://doi.org/10.12980/APJTB.4.201414B448.

Tripathi, Anushree. & Krishna, Misra. (2017). "Molecular Docking : A Structure- Based Drug Designing Approach." *JSciMed Chemistry*, *5* (2), 1042.

Veber, Daniel F., Stephen, R. Johnson., Hung-Yuan, Cheng., Brian, R. Smith., Keith, W. Ward. & Kenneth, D. Kopple. (2002). "Molecular Properties That Influence the Oral Bioavailability of Drug Candidates." *Journal of Medicinal Chemistry*, *45* (12), 2615–23. https://doi.org/10.1021/jm020017n.

Veljkovic, Veljko., Marco, Goeijenbier., Sanja, Glisic., Nevena, Veljkovic., Vladimir, R. Perovic., Milan, Sencanski., Donald, R. Branch. & Slobodan, Paessler. (2015). "In Silico Analysis Suggests Repurposing of Ibuprofen for Prevention and Treatment of EBOLA

Virus Disease." *F1000Research*, *4* (104), 1–9. https://doi.org/
10.12688/f1000research.6436.1.

Vilar, Santiago., Giorgio, Cozza. & Stefano, Moro. (2008). "Medicinal
Chemistry and the Molecular Operating Environment (MOE):
Application of QSAR and Molecular Docking to Drug Discovery."
Current Topics in Medicinal Chemistry, *8* (18), 1555–72. https://
doi.org/10.2174/156802608786786624.

Wang, Xin., Ke, Song., Li, Li. & Lijiang, Chen. (2018). "Structure-Based
Drug Design Strategies and Challenges." *Current Topics in Medicinal
Chemistry*, *18* (12), 998–1006. https://doi.org/10.2174/1568026618666
180813152921.

Watanabe, Shinji., Takeshi, Noda. & Yoshihiro, Kawaoka. (2006).
"Functional Mapping of the Nucleoprotein of Ebola Virus." *Journal of
Virology*, *80* (8), 3743–51. https://doi.org/10.1128/JVI.80.8.3743-
3751.2006.

Wishart, David S. (2005). "Bioinformatics in Drug Development and
Assessment." *Drug Metabolism Reviews*, *37* (2), 279–310. https://
doi.org/10.1081/DMR-55225.

World Health Organization. (2018). "Ebola Virus Disease." 2018. https://
www.who.int/news-room/fact-sheets/detail/ebola-virus-disease.

Yanuar, Arry., Heru, Suhartanto., Abdul, Mun'im., Bram, Hik Anugraha.
& Rezi, Riadhi Syahdi. (2014). "Virtual Screening of Indonesian
Herbal Database as HIV-1 Protease Inhibitor." *Bioinformation*, *10* (2),
52–55. https://doi.org/10.6026/97320630010052.

Yuan, Yuan. (2015). "Possible FDA-Approved Drugs to Treat Ebola Virus
Infection." *Infectious Diseases of Poverty*, *4*, 23. https://doi.
org/10.1186/s40249-015-0055-z.

Zaki, Sherif R., Wun-Ju, Shieh., Patricia, W. Greer., Cynthia, S.
Goldsmith., Tara, Ferebee., Jacques, Katshitshi., Kweteminga Tshioko,
F., et al. (1999). "A Novel Immunohistochemical Assay for the
Detection of Ebola Virus in Skin: Implications for Diagnosis, Spread,
and Surveillance of Ebola Hemorrhagic Fever." *The Journal of
Infectious Diseases*, *179* (s1), S36–47. https://doi.org/10.1086/514319.

INDEX

Related Nova Publications

ZIKA VIRUS SURVEILLANCE, VACCINOLOGY, AND ANTI-ZIKA DRUG DISCOVERY: COMPUTER-ASSISTED STRATEGIES TO COMBAT THE MENACE

EDITORS: Subhash C. Basak, Ph.D., Apurba K. Bhattacharjee, Ph.D., and Ashesh Nandy, Ph.D.

SERIES: Virology Research Progress

BOOK DESCRIPTION: On 1 February 2016, WHO declared that the association of Zika infection with clusters of microcephaly and other neurological disorders constituted a Public Health Emergency of International Concern. Although the severity and number of ZIKV afflicted cases have gone down lately, the public health community worldwide is keeping a watchful eye on it.

SOFTCOVER ISBN: 978-1-53614-970-8
RETAIL PRICE: $82

PARASITOIDS: BIOLOGY, BEHAVIOR AND ECOLOGY

EDITOR: Emily Donnelly

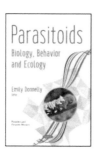

SERIES: Parasites and Parasitic Diseases

BOOK DESCRIPTION: The opening chapter of *Parasitoids: Biology, Behavior and Ecology* discusses the influence of host preference and host specificity in biological control programs and their role in different biological control methods.

SOFTCOVER ISBN: 978-1-53615-197-8
RETAIL PRICE: $82

To see a complete list of Nova publications, please visit our website at www.novapublishers.com